WU 450

KV-700-439

MEDICAL LIBRARY
WATFORD POSTGRADUATE
MEDICAL CENTRE
WATFORD GENERAL HOSPITAL
VICARAGE ROAD
WATFORD WD1 8HB

Functional Orthodontic Appliances

Functional Orthodontic Appliances

K.G. Isaacson FDS, M. Orth, RCS Eng
Consultant Orthodontist,
Oxford Regional Health Authority

R.T. Reed FDS, RCPS Glas, M. Orth, RCS Eng
Consultant Orthodontist,
Wessex Regional Health Authority

C.D. Stephens MDS U. Brist, FDS, RCS Edin,
FDS, M. Orth, RCS Eng
Professor of Child Dental Health,
University of Bristol

MEDICAL LIBRARY
WATFORD POSTGRADUATE
MEDICAL CENTRE
WATFORD GENERAL HOSPITAL
VICARAGE ROAD
WATFORD WD1 8HB

BLACKWELL SCIENTIFIC PUBLICATIONS

OXFORD LONDON

EDINBURGH BOSTON MELBOURNE

© 1990 by
Blackwell Scientific Publications
Editorial offices:
Osney Mead, Oxford OX2 0EL
25 John Street, London WC1N 2BL
23 Ainslie Place, Edinburgh EH3 6AJ
3 Cambridge Center, Suite 208
  Cambridge, Massachusetts 02142, USA
107 Barry Street, Carlton
  Victoria 3053, Australia

All rights reserved. No part of this
publication may be reproduced, stored
in a retrieval system, or transmitted,
in any form or by any means,
electronic, mechanical, photocopying,
recording or otherwise without
the prior permission of the
copyright owner

First published 1990

Set by Setrite Typesetters, Hong Kong;
printed and bound in Great Britain by
William Clowes Limited
Beccles and London

DISTRIBUTORS

Marston Book Services Ltd
PO Box 87
Oxford OX2 0DT
(*Orders*: Tel. 0865 791155
        Fax: 0865 791927
        Telex: 837515)

USA
Year Book Medical Publishers
200 North LaSalle Street
Chicago, Illinois 60601
(*Orders*: Tel: (312) 726−9733)

Canada
The C.V. Mosby Company
5240 Finch Avenue East
Scarborough, Ontario
(*Orders*: Tel: 416 298−1588)

Australia
Blackwell Scientific Publications
(Australia) Pty Ltd
107 Barry Street
Carlton, Victoria 3053
(*Orders*: (03) 347−0300)

British Library
Cataloguing in Publication Data

Isaacson, K.G. (Keith Geoffrey)
  Functional orthodontic appliances.
  1. Man. Orthodontic appliances
  I. Title II. Reed, R. T. III. Stephens, C. D.
  617.6′43′0028

ISBN 0-632-02022-9

Contents

Preface

Functional appliances have been used since the nineteenth century and a wide variety of appliances has been described. Their mode of action varies, but the common feature that separates them from other orthodontic appliances is that the mandible is held away from its rest position by the appliance. Protagonists of functional appliances claim that they use muscular force to redirect facial growth and alter patterns of mandibular development.

The authors have used functional appliances for many years, mainly of the activator type, and whilst appreciating that there is minimal scientific evidence for stimulation of mandibular growth, they have found that the appliances are extremely useful in the correction of skeletal discrepancy in selected patients.

The aim of this book is to explain the action of functional appliances and to give guidance to the selection and clinical management of cases, together with details of some of the more popular appliances.

K.G.I., R.T.R., C.D.S.

Acknowledgements

We wish to thank our many colleagues who have kindly read the manuscript and made constructive suggestions. The Photographic Departments of Bristol Dental School, Basingstoke District Hospital and the Royal Berkshire Hospital have also generously assisted in the preparation of the photographs, and Neil Isaacson helped with the tracings. The cases illustrated in Figs 1.4, 3.4, 5.2, and 5.6 have previously appeared in the *Journal of Clinical Orthodontics*. Finally we would like to thank J.J. Thompson Laboratories for preparing the section on appliance construction.

Chapter 1   The Role of Functional Appliances

The orthodontic world is divided in its appraisal of functional appliances. The protagonists claim that they are able to make changes in the underlying skeletal pattern of the patient and that growth of the mandible may be stimulated by such appliances. They claim the changes that the appliances can make are not merely orthodontic but are orthopaedic in nature. This is in keeping with the functional matrix theory of Moss (1968), who proposes that facial form is modified by function, and that by functional alteration of the resting posture of the mandible alteration of growth is possible.

By contrast the traditional view believes that the form and shape of the facial bones is genetically determined, as is the size of any other bone in the body. Can you make a boy taller by giving him exercises? Does the giraffe's neck become long by reaching for leaves at the top of the tree? Changes are thought to be purely dento-alveolar — in other words, limited to the change that takes place in the alveolar supporting bone when teeth are moved orthodontically.

The truth may be somewhere between these opposing views, and may never be completely resolved because of the complexity of inter-relating factors that give rise to successful treatment. One thing is certain: functional appliances are only of any real advantage when employed in the mouth of a growing child and their effect in adults is undoubtedly restricted to dento-alveolar change, which can be achieved, in our opinion, more satisfactorily with conventional appliances. We do not advise the use of functional appliances in adults.

Terminology may be confusing — some advocate the use of the term *myo-functional* as they consider the muscular reflex action of the facial muscles important in the action of the appliance. In North America they are classified as removable appliances (in contrast to fixed appliances). Within the United Kingdom the term *removable appliance* is restricted to appliances worn in one arch, which carry active spring components.

The authors prefer the term *functional appliance* to cover all those appliances which engage both arches and act principally by holding the mandible away from its normal resting position. It will be apparent that there are functional aspects in almost all (one-arch) removable appliances, in particular the effect of a bite plane or molar capping in altering the relative eruption rates of the molars and incisors. Oral screens and Positioners (which may be used at the end of fixed appliance treatment) are also functional in their effect. The main distinction between functional and removable appliances is that functional appliances act by holding the mandible in a postured position.

Main categories of appliance

The relevance of growth, the mode of action and the management of appliances will be covered in general terms that apply to all kinds of functional appliance. For the purposes of description there are two broad categories of appliance — those that are primarily rigid and made of acrylic, like the Andresen (Fig. 1.1a), and those that are more flexible, incorporating a much greater amount of wire work, exemplified by the function regulator (FR) of Frankel (Fig. 1.1). The action of all appliances is basically similar, although Frankel claims that his appliance is an exercise appliance to enable the patient to develop normal function, and subsequently normal form. The varieties of functional appliance are now legion — and each appliance becomes modified by different operators. Active components may be incorporated, most commonly screws and springs, and labial bows may be used to achieve conventional orthodontic movement of a tooth or groups of teeth.

This is a clinical book and it is the authors' intention to describe some of the more commonly used appliances. Where appliances have eponymous names it may be found that the appliance is not described in its original version. We do not subscribe to the view that unless an appliance is made exactly as originally described, it will not produce the desired changes. It is inevitable that in clinical use such appliances are constantly being modified and improved. Furthermore, specific considerations of an individual malocclusion may determine a particular alteration in design.

Historical background

The first types of functional appliance were developed from the use of removable appliances incorporating bite planes. Catalan in Spain in the late 19th century used an inclined anterior bite plane with the intention of causing the mandible to be postured forward in the hope that this would cause a 'jumping of the bite' and stimulate growth of the mandible, thus changing a Class II buccal segment relationship into Class I.

Robin (1902) was the first to describe an appliance which was specifically designed to act on the maxillary and mandibular arches

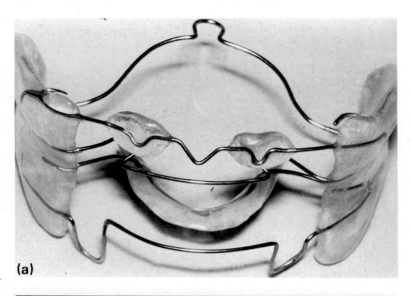

(a)

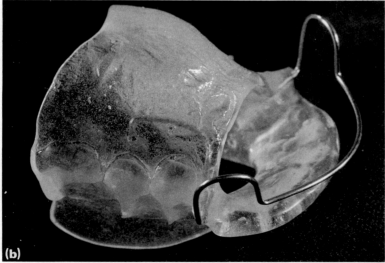

(b)

Fig. 1.1 (a) A Frankel appliance; (b) an Andresen appliance.

simultaneously. The appliance was intended to expand both the upper and lower arches and to bring the mandible forwards. The significance of the appliance was perhaps lost amongst his view that malocclusion could give rise to all sorts of maladies.

Rogers (1918) was an advocate of muscle training exercises with the use of functional appliances to encourage correct growth of the dental structures. Although these did not find favour for very long they drew attention to the importance of muscle activity and growth. Andresen was developing his appliance at about the same time as Robin was experimenting with his monobloc. Andresen, however, was completely unaware of Robin's work. The original Andresen appliance was developed from an upper removable appliance initially incorporating bite planes with lingual extensions. It was designed as a passive retaining appliance to be worn during long summer vacations in Norway when fixed appliances were removed because they could not be adequately supervised. Andresen (1939) found to his surprise that the malocclusions actually improved during the holiday period and developed the appliance to enhance these changes and to be used as an independent appliance. Other workers who have done much to advance the development of functional appliances are Haupl, Bimler, Harvold, Grossman and Frankel and they have developed appliances which have different characteristics. However, all have one aspect in common: they deliberately hold the mandible away from its natural resting posture.

Current and future use

Functional appliances are not used as much as they could be in the UK. Indeed until recently less than 1% of the cases approved for treatment within the National Health Service were for functional appliance treatment. Perhaps this has partly been due to a lack of understanding of the appliances themselves and may be seen against the background of argument and counter-argument concerning their mode of action, some clinicians remaining to be convinced of their effectiveness. However, in the British Isles the incidence of crowding is high, uncrowded arches (for which the functional appliances were originally intended) are rarely seen and therefore functional appliances have had less of a following here than elsewhere in Europe. In North America fixed appliances have always been extensively employed in the treatment of all malocclusions and until the late 1970s the use of functional appliances has been even less favoured than in Europe.

Of all the functional appliances the Andresen appliance is still the most well known, but because of its tendency to procline the lower labial segment its use has been confined largely to those cases where there is space in the lower arch. This ensures that any post-treatment relapse of this unintended movement is not accompanied by incisor crowding (Walther 1967, Tulley & Campbell 1960). Functional appliances, therefore, have been used for cases with uncrowded and well-aligned arches (Fig. 1.2). Nowadays they enjoy a wider application and are increasingly used in both extraction and non-extraction cases.

Empirically it has been found that proclination of the lower labial segment for either the relief of crowding or the reduction of an increased overjet is unstable in the long term. The principle of maintaining the labio-lingual position of the lower incisor crowns (Mills 1966) has long been accepted in the UK as a sound basis for orthodontic treatment with removable appliances. The authors support this view, although they accept that with fixed appliance techniques it is sometimes possible to alter permanently the labio-lingual position of the lower incisors. It is acknowledged that any type of functional appliance may produce some proclination of the lower labial segment and all users should attempt, by careful design and management, to avoid this possibility. Ideally any change in the position of the lower labial segment should be identified at the end of treatment by means of cephalometric radiography (Fig. 1.3).

Interceptive treatment

Some clinicians recognize and treat aberrant facial growth patterns at an early age, and claim that appliances are best at stimulating growth during the early mixed dentition stage. Although there is considerable natural growth occurring at this stage we believe that there is no overall benefit in such early treatment. This view will disappoint many, but is based on much experience with the appliances. In most young patients there is a limit to the amount of co-operation that is available. Three years seems to be an upper limit and it is preferable to keep treatment time to within a 2-year period if possible. When treatment is commenced before the age of 10, the final result cannot be achieved until the permanent dentition is established (Fig. 1.4). Although primarily discussing conventional appliances, Fletcher (1958) has demonstrated the problems of early treatment. He found that the younger the patient at the start of treatment the longer the treatment time.

We consider that, apart from exceptional cases, the child of 7–10 years is not likely to be sufficiently mature to cope with the wearing of loose-fitting, bulky appliances, particularly when this may be required during school and social activities. In gross Class II division 1 cases occasionally there may be sufficient motivation for a patient to wear an appliance to reduce an overjet, and this can have both social and preventative advantages, but, in general, the experience of the authors is that severe cases can be treated satisfactorily during the pubertal growth spurt.

A major change in our approach to the use of functional appliances has been their application to cases where crowding necessitates premolar extractions. Another advantage is the ability to utilize fixed appliances both simultaneously, and following treatment with a functional appliance. For example, it is possible to improve a skeletal discrepancy between the maxilla and mandible and then to carry out precise positioning of the occlusion with fixed appliances at a later stage. Even removable appliances can be used subsequent to functional appliance treatment where premolars have been extracted. Having improved a skeletal discrepancy, other appliances may then be used to complete treatment.

Commitment

The importance of a practitioner's involvement with the patient and the appliance is never greater than when using functional appliances. The wearing of appliances requires dedication from the patient, and to instil the necessary commitment to co-operation, it is essential that the operator is fully conversant with the appliance and its capabilities. This presents problems in chairside training where clinical instruction to a professional colleague can easily influence the patient in the belief that their treatment may in some way be experimental and as a result the necessary co-operation is not achieved. This factor is, we are certain, a very real one in the rejection of functional appliances, not only by the patient but also by those instructed in their use. A polyclinic atmosphere with changing staff is an inappropriate place in which to carry out such treatment and may largely explain why studies conducted in hospital departments have shown limited success (Cohen 1981). A one-to-one relationship between practitioner and patient, with an understanding nursing and reception staff, is a formula for success in such treatment.

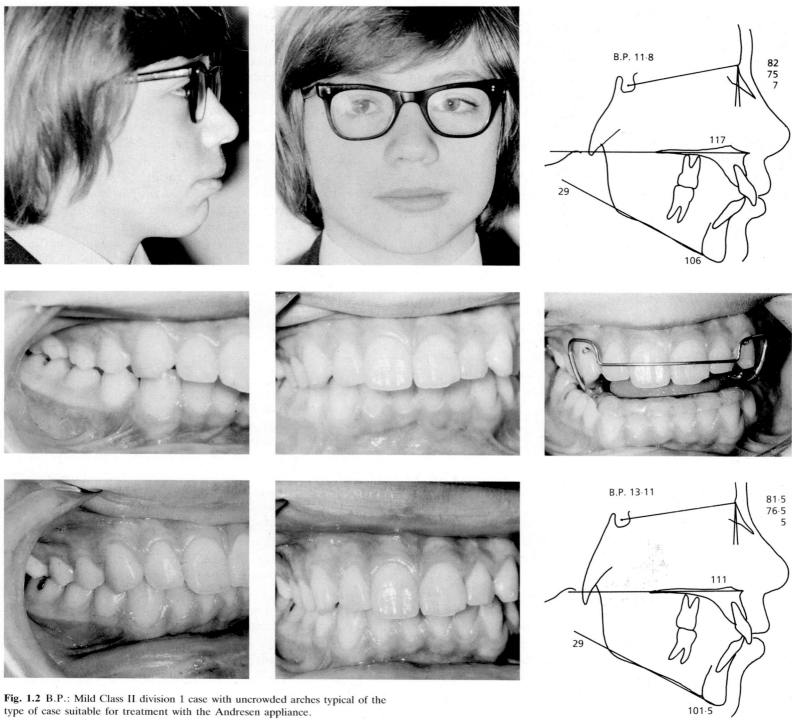

Fig. 1.2 B.P.: Mild Class II division 1 case with uncrowded arches typical of the type of case suitable for treatment with the Andresen appliance.

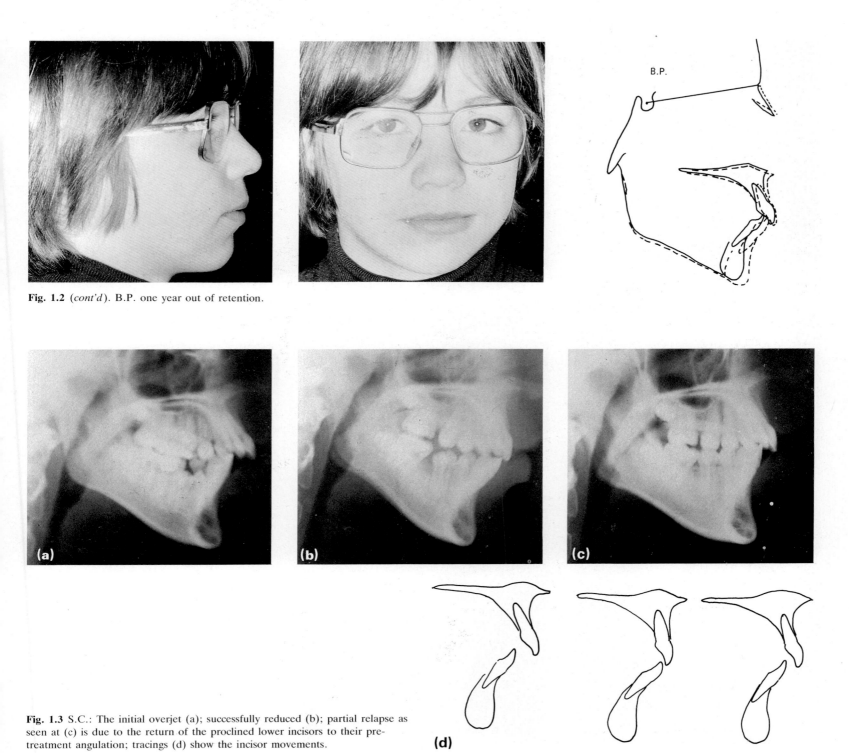

Fig. 1.2 (*cont'd*). B.P. one year out of retention.

Fig. 1.3 S.C.: The initial overjet (a); successfully reduced (b); partial relapse as seen at (c) is due to the return of the proclined lower incisors to their pre-treatment angulation; tracings (d) show the incisor movements.

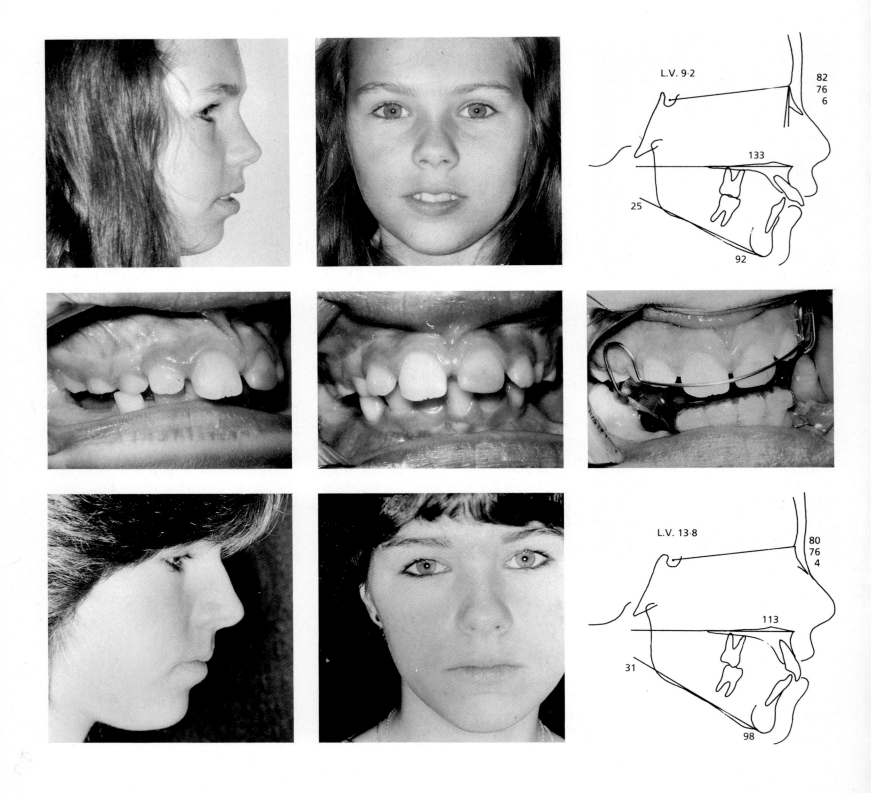

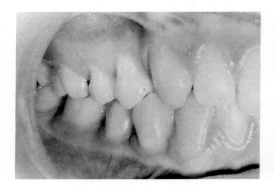 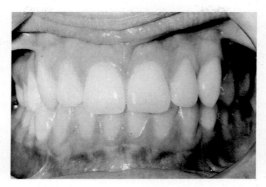 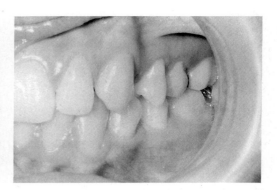

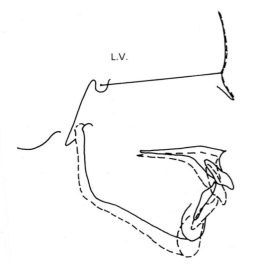

Fig. 1.4 L.V.: Repeated fracture of the left central incisor required early overjet reduction. The overjet was fully reduced in 6 months while still in the mixed dentition. Retention was continued until the premolars had erupted 4½ years later.

Advantages and disadvantages of functional appliances

Despite the controversy that surrounds the use of functional appliances their uses and limitations can be clearly defined. These are summarized in Table 1.1.

Table 1.1 Advantages and disadvantages of functional appliances

Advantages	Disadvantages
Utilize the growth potential of the dental arches to a maximum, and can achieve a better improvement in the profile than conventional appliances	Precise detailing of tooth position not possible
Treatment can be commenced in the mixed dentition stage, and can be effective during the pubertal growth spurt where this occurs before full eruption of premolars and canines	Variable response in the post-pubertal patient and ineffective in the adult
Ideal for the treatment of uncrowded Class II division 1 malocclusions	Crowded cases more difficult to manage. Incisor rotations are a contra-indication to treatment
Effective at vertical control of increased overbites	Precise correction of inter-incisal angulation not possible
Minimal chairside time with less frequent adjustment	Totally dependent upon patient co-operation
Economic way of delivering care to a larger number of patients	To achieve high standards fixed appliances are usually required for final detailing of the occlusion

References

Andresen, V. & Haupl, K. (1939) *Funktions Kieferorthopadie*. Meusser, Leipzig.

Cohen, A. (1981) Class II division I malocclusion treated by Andresen appliance. *British Journal of Orthodontics*, **8**, 159.

Fletcher, G.C.T. (1958) The age factor in orthodontics. *Transactions of the British Society for the Study of Orthodontics*, **31**.

Mills, J.R.E. (1966) The stability of the lower labial segment. *Dental Practitioner and Dental Record*, **18**, 293.

Moss, M. (1968) The primacy of functional matrices in orofacial growth. *Transactions of the British Society for the Study of Orthodontics*, 107.

Robin, P. (1902) Observations sur un nouvel appareil de redressment. *Review of Stomatology*, **9**, 423.

Rogers, A.P. (1918) Exercises for the development of the face. *Dental Cosmos*, **60**, 857.

Tulley, W.J. & Campbell, A.C. (1960) *A Manual of Practical Orthodontics*. J. Wright, Bristol.

Walther, D.P. (1967) *Orthodontic Notes*. J. Wright, Bristol.

Further reading

Graber, T.M. & Neumann, B. (1985) *Removable Orthodontic Appliance* 2nd edn, p. 55. W.B. Saunders, Philadelphia.

Schmuth, G.P.F. (1983) Milestones in the development of functional appliances. *American Journal of Orthodontics*, **84**, 48.

Chapter 2   The Importance of Growth

The relevance of growth

In order to appreciate the changes which may be brought about by functional appliances it is necessary to have an understanding of the normal mechanisms of growth. The nature of the human growth pattern and particularly the pubertal growth spurt as it affects the face are considered in this chapter.

Dentofacial development

The growth of the facial skeleton is complex and has been studied in the human largely by serial radiographic techniques. The Bolton Study, work at the Centre for Human Dentofacial Growth at Ann Arbor and the Burlington Study have been notable North American contributions to the study of dentofacial growth whilst in Europe the implant studies of Björk and Skieller have been pre-eminent.

Anatomically the skull may be divided into the neurocranium, which houses the brain, and the viscerocranium or facial skeleton, which contains the jaws and teeth and is enveloped in the oro-masticatory musculature to form the face. Between these two and shared by them is the cranial base which develops from the cartilaginous chondrocranium of the foetus. Early in life centres of ossification develop within this cartilage which, as a result, is gradually replaced by bone.

The orthodontist is used to looking at the skull in lateral projection on radiographs. For this reason, and because midline structures stand out clearly in lateral skull films, the cranial base is usually defined in terms of mid-sagittal structures extending from basion to nasion (Fig. 2.1).

The cranial base may be divided into an anterior part, extending from nasion to sella, and a posterior part from sella to basion. The upper facial skeleton is attached beneath the anterior part whilst the mandible is indirectly joined to the posterior part via the temporal bone. The anterior and posterior parts of the cranial base form a marked angle at the sella, the cranial base angle. Usually this is around 125 degrees and variations in the angle have a profound effect on the relationship of the jaws. A rather obtuse angle will cause the mandible to be positioned posterior to

the maxilla and will make a skeletal two-jaw relationship more likely (Fig. 2.2). The cranial floor has been described by Enlow & McNamara (1973) as the template on which the face develops.

In the child, two important sites of growth remain within the

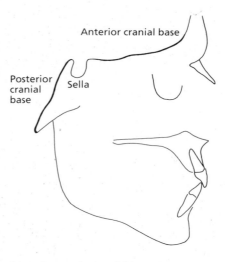

Fig. 2.1 The anterior and posterior cranial bases.

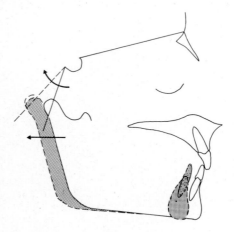

Fig. 2.2 Variation in the cranial base angle (between the posterior and anterior cranial base) influences the relative antero-posterior position of the glenoid fossa and thus the antero-posterior position of the mandible.

cranial base and are responsible for its growth within the orthodontic period. These are the spheno-ethmoidal and the spheno-occipital synchondroses (Fig. 2.3). Growth at the former ceases at about 7 years (Roche & Lewis 1976) whilst at the latter it continues until puberty.

In studies of dentofacial growth during orthodontic treatment the anterior cranial base (usually defined in terms of the sella—nasion line) is used as a reference plane upon which to superimpose serial radiographs. This is because research has shown the anterior cranial base to be relatively stable after growth of the brain and growth at the spheno-ethmoidal suture ceases at around 7 years. However the nasion continues to grow forwards until facial growth ceases and so it has become customary to superimpose upon sella alone but keep the two sella—nasion lines coincidental.

The upper face

The face is usually described as growing downwards and forwards relative to the brain and cranial base (Fig. 2.4). Implant studies have shown there to be considerable remodelling of individual bones of the upper face and this downwards translation should be regarded as an overall effect which is produced by:

1 Growth at the circum-maxillary sutures.

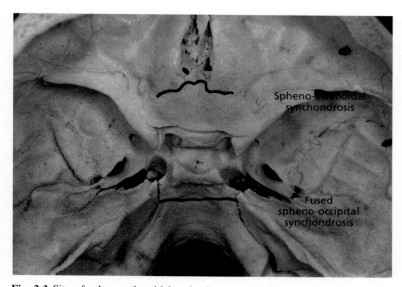

Fig. 2.3 Site of spheno-ethmoidal and spheno-occipital synchondroses.

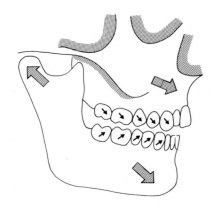

Fig. 2.4 The upper face grows downwards and forwards relative to the cranial base.

2 Change in the relationship of bones one to another at these sutures.

3 Increase in size of individual bones by surface apposition and resorption.

4 Dento-alveolar growth.

Sutural growth plays a significant role in early growth. The fibrous joints, which form the sutures of the face, are now believed to be adaptive sites with little if any capacity for independent growth. Some underlying growth-promoting force must occur to displace the maxilla downwards and forwards.

Various hypotheses have been advanced:

(a) growth of the nasal septum (Scott 1953);

(b) growth of the orbit;

(c) functional demands of surrounding systems—the Functional Matrix concept (Moss 1968); and

(d) the action of myofibroblasts at the sutures (Azuma *et al.* 1975) which because of the orientation of the sutures would produce both a downward and forward translation of the maxilla.

At the present time no one mechanism seems any more likely than any other and indeed all may contribute to the total effect.

Whilst the naso-maxillary complex is translated forward and downward as a result of growth at sutures, post-natal growth in height, breadth and length of the maxilla is largely the result of alveolar growth and associated surface apposition. During this period there is also highly co-ordinated remodelling of the nasal floor and the floor of the antrum. The overall contribution made by these various mechanisms to vertical upper face growth from

4 years to adulthood have recently been quantified by implant studies as follows:

1 Sutural lowering of the maxilla: 11.2 mm (range 9.5−13.5 mm).

2 Growth in height of the alveolar processes: 14.6 mm (range 11.5−17.5 mm).

3 Resorptive lowering of the nasal floor: 4.6 mm (range 1.5−7.5 mm).

So well is the overall shape of the maxilla preserved throughout growth that on serial lateral skull radiographs the maxilla appears to undergo a steady downwards and forwards progression. For this reason many clinicians in the past have been led to believe that superimposition on pre- and post-treatment maxillary outlines will reveal the tooth movements which orthodontic treatment has achieved in the upper arch.

Growth of the mandible

At birth, the mandible is a curved bar of bone with a very poorly developed coronoid process and an obtuse flattened gonial angle. The condylar cartilage, which is large and 'carrot-shaped', is rapidly converted to bone until it is only a cap of cartilage covering the head of the condyle. By the end of the first year of life growth at the symphysis has almost ceased and mandibular growth thereafter is achieved by:

1 Appositional growth at the surface of the condylar cartilage.

2 Surface deposition of bone, notably at the posterior border of the ramus and on the outer surfaces of the body.

3 Dento-alveolar growth.

The role of the condylar cartilage in post-natal mandibular growth is very relevant to orthodontic treatment, but unfortunately is the subject of much controversy. Some of this has arisen because the mandible has been viewed merely as a curved long bone with the condylar cartilage likened to an epiphyseal plate. However, although they are situated at the end of the shaft of a long bone the epiphyseal cartilages are not located directly beneath an articular surface. There is always a certain amount of bone between the epiphyseal plate and the articular cartilage on a long bone (Fig. 2.5). In the mandible, on the other hand, the condylar cartilage abuts directly on to the fibrocartilage which forms the articular surface. This is not the only point of difference. Most authors now agree that the condylar cartilage differs from other primary cartilages in that it grows by apposition rather than

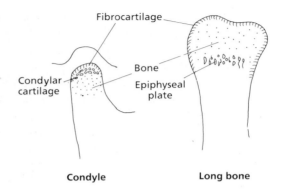

Fig. 2.5 The differing locations of cartilage in the mandibular condyle and epiphysis of a long bone.

interstitially. In this respect it may be likened to periosteum and may therefore be more susceptible to modification by external forces than an epiphyseal plate.

Some work has shown that the condyle has an independent growth potential. Others have found that this is lost in a non-functional environment and feel that the condyle merely responds to the demands of the functional matrix. Whatever the controlling mechanism, growth at the condyle is necessary for normal mandibular growth.

A further factor to be appreciated when studying facial growth is the growth rotation which takes place in the enlarging maxilla and more especially the growing mandible. Björk, in a number of papers, has shown that in most individuals there is an upwards and forwards rotation of the mandibular corpus (Fig. 2.6) but that this is to a very large extent masked by remodelling at its inferior and posterior margins. This rotation has a significant influence on the vertical growth of the maxilla, on the posterior and anterior lower face height and on the overbite. Occasionally backwards rotation patterns are seen which tend to be associated with an anterior open bite. Not only is the degree and direction of rotation important but also the location of its axis. This centre of growth rotation may lie anywhere between the lower incisal edges and the molar region.

Growth in stature

All orthodontists should have an understanding of the process of human growth and development. It might be assumed that human growth occurs in a linear fashion from birth until full adult size is achieved and such a concept would be reinforced by cross-sectional studies. If groups of children of the same age are measured and the mean heights of each compared with groups of differing ages, any variation in individual growth rates tends to be disguised. If, however, individuals are measured over a period of time it becomes apparent that the rate of growth is not constant. These changes are seen on a graph which plots the height of the individual against the age. This is described as a distance curve

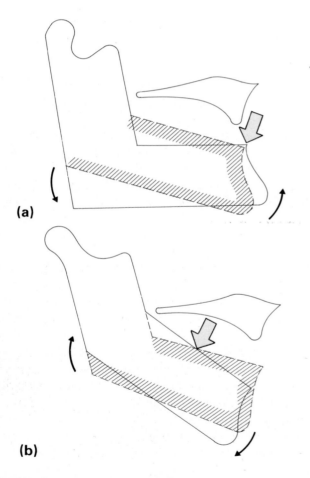

Fig. 2.6 Mandibular growth rotation may take place either about the lower incisor edges, the premolars, or the molars (Björk & Skieller 1972). (a) In the diagram, forward rotation is shown taking place at about the lower incisal edges. (b) An example of downwards and backwards mandibular rotation taking place at the premolars is shown.

(Fig. 2.7). Quite significant changes in the rate of growth (growth spurts) are represented by very slight changes in the inclination of the graph. However, it can be seen from these curves that there is a distinct difference between individuals with regard to the periods at which pubertal growth increase occurs and the time at which growth is complete. In particular there is a significant difference between the sexes. The classic work on growth and stature has been carried out by Tanner & Whitehouse at the Institute of Child Health in London (1976).

In order to demonstrate the varying rates of human growth more clearly, it is better that the data are presented as a velocity curve, which is obtained by plotting the rate of growth at any given time against the age (Fig. 2.8). There are times of relatively slow growth and other times of more rapid growth. The greatest rate of growth occurs during the first year of life, the rate then declines rapidly until about five or six years of age when the decline in growth rate levels out, remaining at a fairly constant rate until a second period of increased growth occurs at puberty. The velocity curves also clearly demonstrate the difference between individuals and particularly the difference between the sexes.

The maximum rate of growth which occurs during adolescence is called the *peak height velocity* (PHV). In boys, the average age at which the PHV is reached is 14 years. There is, however, a wide variation and two standard deviations are equivalent to plus or minus two years (Fig. 2.9). In girls, PHV occurs at an average age of 12 years with a similar standard deviation. There is evidence that, in a significant number of females, there is no distinct pubertal growth spurt (Tanner & Whitehouse 1979). The age at which growth in stature ceases shows a similar variation and sexual differentiation. There is a very considerable individual variation at which specific growth milestones are reached.

Woodside (1973) and others in Toronto, using data from the Burlington growth study, have been able to demonstrate that very similar patterns can be seen in the rate of growth of the facial bones and in particular of the mandible. Distance and velocity growth curves can be drawn for the mandibular length of both sexes which closely mimic the graphs produced by Tanner & Whitehouse demonstrating the growth in human stature (Figs 2.10 and 2.11). Once again the most striking feature of Woodside's study is the great difference between the sexes: on average the peak of the pubertal growth spurt occurs two years earlier in girls than boys. Although these studies are of considerable interest, it is difficult to make practical use of such data

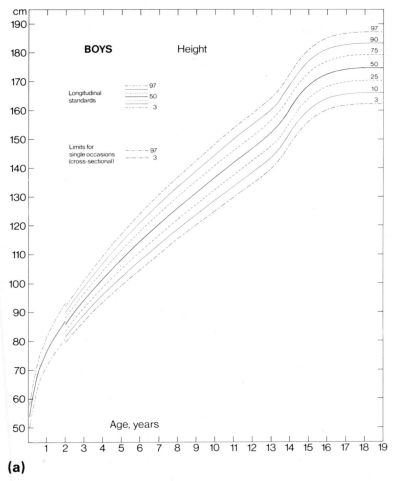

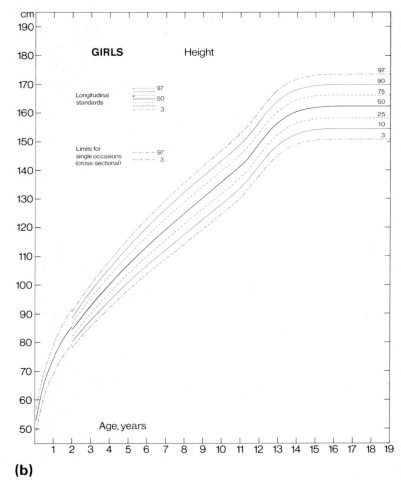

Fig. 2.7 Growth in stature — a distance curve: (a) males, (b) females.

when determining the possible onset of a period of rapid growth for a given individual, because of the wide range of variation. In patients who exhibit rapid and favourable facial growth, sagittal changes can occur with remarkable rapidity. On the other hand if the patient is undergoing little or no facial growth the treatment changes are so small as to make the clinician suspect that his patient is failing to achieve a satisfactory period of appliance wear. It is therefore important to make some attempt to monitor the growth during treatment as well as to obtain from the patient a diary of daily wear. In this way encouragement or admonishment can be given as appropriate.

Although it has yet to be supported by objective data the authors are of the opinion that there is also a relationship between growth and relapse. All orthodontic treatment is liable to relapse to some extent but generally relapse of functional appliance treatment is quite rare. This may be because the rate of change tends to slow down as treatment progresses. As night-time wear of functional appliances presents little problem for the patient, the period of retention tends to be rather longer than in conventional orthodontic treatment.

Occasionally quite a significant increase in overjet is seen in a treated Class II division 1 case many months after the withdrawal of appliances. In the small number of cases in which this has occurred we have observed the following features:

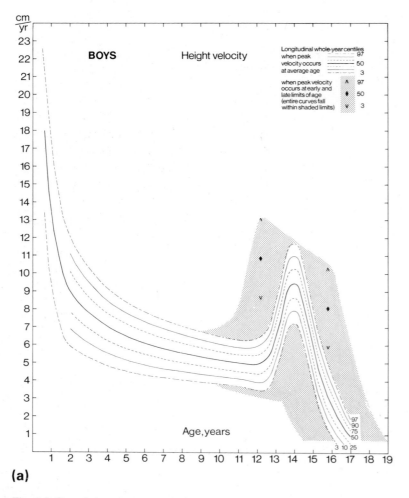

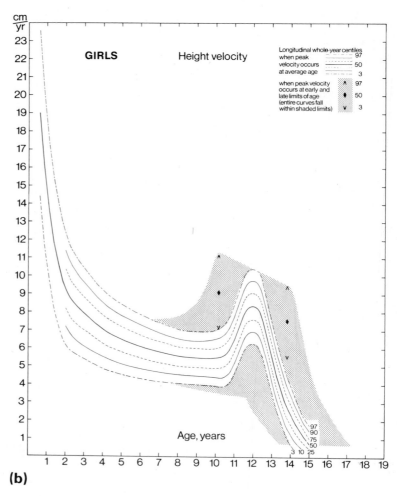

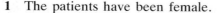

Fig. 2.8 Growth in stature—a velocity curve: (a) males, (b) females.

1 The patients have been female.

2 All entered a marked late growth spurt (as recorded by stature measurements) following the withdrawal of appliances.

3 Where treatment has been carried out by re-introduction of functional appliances, and where retention has been maintained until growth in stature has ceased, a stable result has been achieved (Fig. 2.12).

It can be seen why such cases are rare. Firstly, we always attempt to match treatment to include the pubertal growth period. Secondly, where this is not the case it is either because there has been no growth spurt, or more commonly because the patient is already well into the growth spurt at the time of referral. Why this phenomenon has not yet been observed in males is difficult to explain. Perhaps a tendency to relapse is masked by the greater mandibular growth seen in the male during puberty.

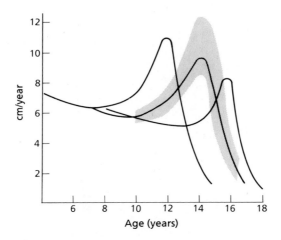

Fig. 2.9 Variation in the time of peak height velocity. The peaks represent two standard deviations either side of the mean for males. 95% of the population will lie within these limits (12–16 years).

The prediction of the timing of facial pubertal growth

Although changes in stature may be easily recorded, and have been widely reported, longitudinal studies of facial growth around puberty are fairly rare and usually involve radiographic studies of limited numbers of subjects. Generally the correlation between timing and amounts of facial and statural growth have been difficult to establish. Bishara *et al.* (1981) conclude that timing of changes in mandibular size and in its relationship to the upper face are not closely correlated and therefore not accurately predictable from recordings of stature. On the other hand vertical changes of the face (which appear to be greatly influenced by functional appliances) occur at rates which reflect statural growth (Baume, Buschang & Weinstein 1983).

It would obviously be best if the rate of facial growth could be

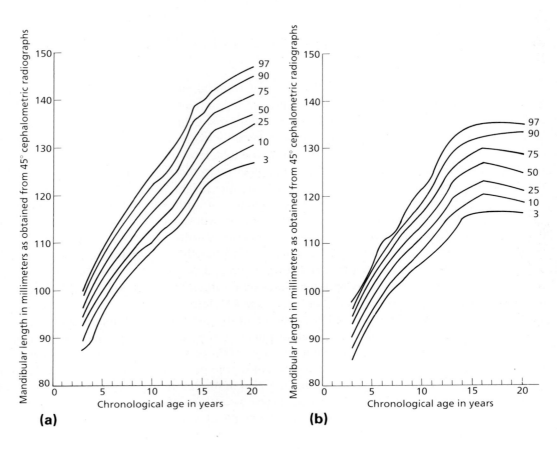

Fig. 2.10 Mandibular distance growth curves: (a) male, (b) female (after Woodside 1973).

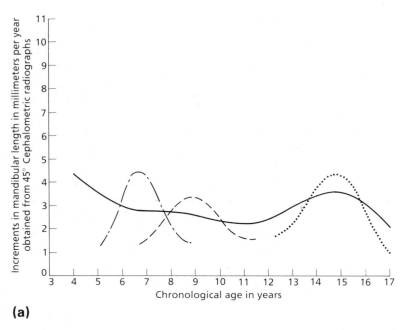

(a)

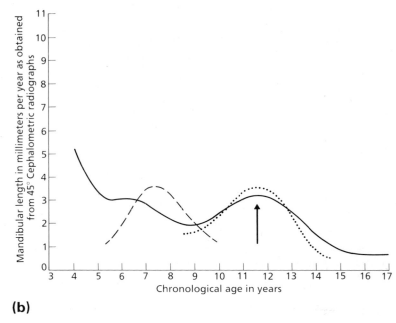

(b)

Fig. 2.11 Mandibular velocity growth curves: (a) male, (b) female (after Woodside 1973).

monitored directly, but the rates of change even when at their greatest are quite small and require a very precise measurement technique. At present only serial radiography offers this degree of precision and cephalometric radiographs at 4-monthly intervals cannot be contemplated because of the unreasonable level of radiation involved. Estimates of facial growth velocity are therefore generally made indirectly from records of standing height.

One of the problems when using the rate of change of stature to obtain an insight into the timing of the adolescent growth spurt is that several records are required in order to construct a growth velocity curve. It is then possible to determine retrospectively when the peak of growth occurred. Prediction is more difficult. Sullivan (1983), using growth velocity templates and a minimum of four measurements of stature taken at 4-monthly intervals starting no later than 10 years of age, has shown that it is possible to predict, with limited accuracy, the peak of pubertal growth in stature one year in advance of this event. In boys, 95% of such predictions will lie within the range 22 months before the peak to 2 months after the peak. For girls the limits are 25 months before the peak to 3 months after the peak. Provided such measurements can be made early enough these predictions will be of value.

Where this is not possible a considerable part of potential treatment time may be lost whilst these measurements are made. For this reason some authorities suggest treatment should be instituted as early as possible, particularly where sagittal discrepancies are marked. The point has also been made that growth only occurs once and the less that remains to take place the less will be the clinician's influence on its outcome. Such advice ignores the reality that patients rarely tolerate more than two or three years treatment and so an excessively early orthodontic intervention runs the risk that the patient will discontinue treatment before the period of maximum growth is fully utilized.

Another approach has been to rely upon ossification events in 'hand wrist' radiographs to identify changes thought to preceed the onset of puberty. Early work indicated that the adductor sesamoid of the thumb always ossified before puberty. It is now recognized that, taken by itself, the sesamoid does not provide a reliable indication. More recently, attempts have been made to use other ossification events to predict peak height velocity. Unfortunately, even when serial hand wrist films have been examined by experts it has been found that the uncertainty of prediction of peak height velocity is generally large and they are of limited value for this purpose unless the child's physical development is markedly advanced or retarded (Houston, Miller & Tanner 1979).

One final general point should be made and that is that the commencement of orthodontic treatment is often dictated by the stage of dental development, although this is less so with functional appliances which can be used before premolar eruption.

The prediction of facial growth

Even if the timing of periods of rapid facial growth can be predicted within broad limits this information would be of much greater value if the future amount of growth could be predicted. For example very occasionally a case is seen in which a skeletal Class 2 sagittal jaw relationship corrects to a large degree without treatment. In such a case treatment might well be inappropriate. Can such cases be predicted? It has to be emphasized that significant spontaneous change in sagittal jaw relationship is extremely rare and generally jaw relationships remain remarkably constant from the time the incisors have erupted until the end of growth. For this reason many clinicians run their practices on the basis that there will be no change in jaw relationship during the period of orthodontic treatment. Whilst such a working hypothesis is satisfactory for the average case it is inadequate for the extremes of variation.

One way of attempting to arrive at a more satisfactory prediction of future growth is to add growth increments to the face as it appears at the time of examination. Such values, adjusted for age and sex, may be drawn in on the patient's cephalometric tracing. It is of course important to know the direction in which this growth will take place and once again only an average value can be taken. Clearly a much better estimate can be made for the patient if serial skull radiographs, taken over a number of years, are available. It is then possible to say whether the patient's facial growth to date has been following an average path. Unfortunately, it is unusual to have such records unless the patient is referred particularly early.

For the patient who has no early cephalometric data the only refinement to the general principle of adding average increments to the cephalometric tracing is to define more closely the population from which the incremental data are derived. For example it is obviously erroneous to add values derived from male Caucasians to the cephalometric records of a female patient of Afro-Caribbean

origin and it is generally accepted that data must be comparable at least for age, sex and race to serve any useful purpose. It would also be an improvement to use data obtained from patients of similar genetic background. For example it would be preferable to use English data derived from patients having Class II malocclusions when attempting to predict the facial growth of an English child with a Class II division 1 malocclusion. With the advent of computers such additions can be carried out rapidly with the aid of a digitizer and plotter. It must be remembered that the idea of an 'individualized' growth prediction remains limited by the need to use average values which can never identify those whose growth patterns are at all unusual.

Some authors have suggested making an attempt to classify the patient according to the underlying growth pattern. It is difficult to make this decision without having serial records of the particular patient and even so there is no absolute certainty that the direction of facial growth will remain constant. Nevertheless, it may be helpful to identify those showing marked extremes of growth pattern (horizontal or vertical) and to select appropriate data, always assuming these are available.

For those who do not have cephalometric radiographs available, facial growth prediction is impossible. It is then impossible to eliminate unusual growth patterns as a possible cause of treatment failure although when orthodontic treatment is started in the late mixed/early permanent dentition 75% of facial growth has, on average, already occurred.

The measurement of standing height

From what has already been said the reader may be in doubt as to the usefulness of any form of measurement which attempts to monitor a patient's general growth as a means to improving orthodontic treatment.

The availability of a growth curve has the following advantages:
1 It may help to avoid starting functional treatment at a time when growth is at the pre-pubertal minimum.
2 It enables retention to be continued until the peak of facial growth is likely to have been passed. This may be especially important for female patients.
3 It will identify patients whose growth is markedly atypical: for example, patients with undetected organic disease or growth hormone deficiency (Hathorn 1986).

Obviously, records of standing height should start as early as

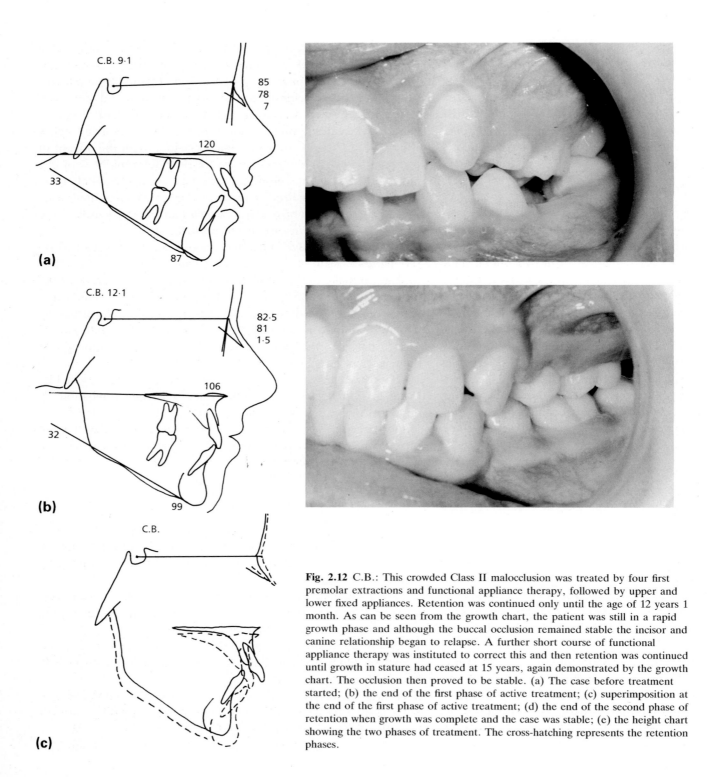

Fig. 2.12 C.B.: This crowded Class II malocclusion was treated by four first premolar extractions and functional appliance therapy, followed by upper and lower fixed appliances. Retention was continued only until the age of 12 years 1 month. As can be seen from the growth chart, the patient was still in a rapid growth phase and although the buccal occlusion remained stable the incisor and canine relationship began to relapse. A further short course of functional appliance therapy was instituted to correct this and then retention was continued until growth in stature had ceased at 15 years, again demonstrated by the growth chart. The occlusion then proved to be stable. (a) The case before treatment started; (b) the end of the first phase of active treatment; (c) superimposition at the end of the first phase of active treatment; (d) the end of the second phase of retention when growth was complete and the case was stable; (e) the height chart showing the two phases of treatment. The cross-hatching represents the retention phases.

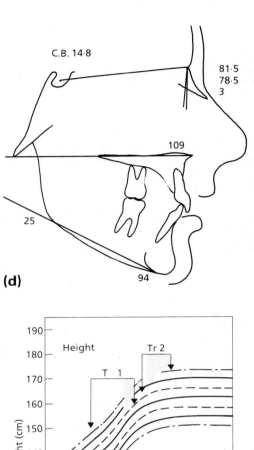

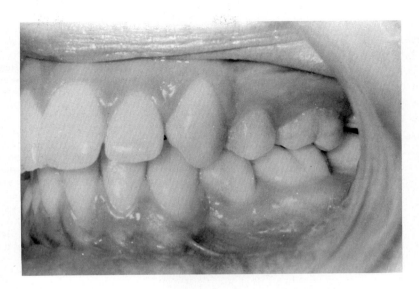

(d)

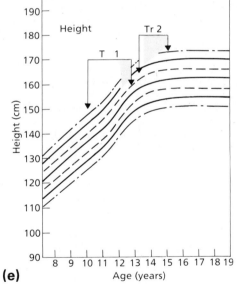

(e)

Fig. 2.12 (*cont'd*)

possible and be made using a reliable stadiometer. Although the Harpenden Stadiometer (Fig. 2.13; available from Holtain, Crosswell, Crymych, Dyfed, SA41 3UF) is probably an unreasonable investment for even a specialist orthodontic practitioner, there are now cheaper stadiometers available which give adequate precision if used carefully (Microtoise height gauge, available

from CMS Weighing Equipment, 18 Camden High Street, London NW1 OJA).

Records should be taken at each visit by the same person and preferably at the same time of day. Shoes should be removed and the patient encouraged to stretch to their maximum height by applying firm digital pressure beneath both mastoid processes.

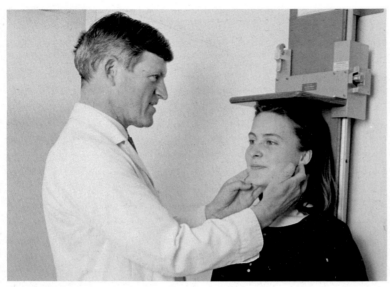

Fig. 2.13 A Harpenden stadiometer.

Each measurement should be repeated and care taken to avoid transposing digits when recording the measurement. Growth charts are now available with a bimonthly scale which is more useful in clinical practice than the more usual decimal year (*Castlemead Publications Height Charts*).

The authors believe that despite their limitations serial stature measurements should be taken of all young orthodontic patients, especially those who are likely to undergo treatment with functional appliances.

References

Azuma, A., Enlow, D.H., Fredrickson, R.G. & Gaston, R.G. (1975) A myofibroblastic basis for the physical forces that produce tooth drift and eruption, skeletal displacement at sutures and periosteal migration. In: MacNamara, J.A. Jr (ed.) *Determinants of mandibular function and growth*. Monograph No. 4, Craniofacial Growth Series. Center for Human Growth and Development, Ann Arbor, Michigan.

Baume, R.M., Buschang, P.H. & Weinstein, S. (1983) Stature, head height and growth of the vertical face. *American Journal of Orthodontics*, **83**, 477.

Bishara, S.E., Jamison, J.E., Peterson, L.C. & DeKock, W.H. (1981) Longitudinal changes in standing height and mandibular parameters between the ages of 8 and 17 years. *American Journal of Orthodontics*, **80**, 115.

Björk, A. & Skieller, V. (1972) Facial development and tooth eruption — an implant study at the age of puberty. *American Journal of Orthodontics*, **62**, 339.

Castlemead Publications Height Charts, reference 11AM and 12AB. Castlemead Publications, Creaseys of Hertford, Castlemead, Hertford, SG14 1LH.

Enlow, D.H. & McNamara, J. Jr (1973) The neurocranial basis for facial form and pattern. *Angle Orthodontist*, **43**, 256.

Hathorn, I.S. (1986) The value of height records in orthodontics. *British Journal of Orthodontics*, **13**, 119.

Houston, W.J.B., Miller, J.C. & Tanner, J.M., (1979) Prediction of the timing of the adolescent growth spurt from ossification events in hand-wrist films. *British Journal of Orthodontics*, **6**, 145.

Moss, M.L. (1968) The primacy of functional matrices in oro-facial growth. *Dental Practitioner and Dental Record*, **19**, 65.

Roche, A.F. & Lewis, A.B. (1976) Later growth changes in the cranial base. In: Bosma, J.F. (ed.) *Symposium on the development of the basicranium*. National Institute of Health, Bethesda.

Scott, J.H. (1953) The cartilage of the nasal septum. *British Dental Journal*, **95**, 37.

Sullivan, P.G. (1983) Prediction of the pubertal growth spurt. *European Journal of Orthodontics*, **5**, 189.

Tanner, J.M. & Whitehouse, R.H., (1976) Clinical longitudinal standards for height and weight. *Archives of Diseases in Childhood*, **51**, 170.

Woodside, D.G. (1973) Some effects of Activator treatment on the mandible and midface. *Transactions of the European Orthodontic Society*, 443.

Further reading

Björk, A. & Skieller, V. (1977) Growth of the maxilla as revealed radiographically by the implant method. *British Journal of Orthodontics*, **4**, 53.

Broadbent, B.H. & Golden, W.H. (1975) *Bolton standards of Dento-Facial Growth*. Mosby, St Louis.

Carlson, D.S. & Ribbens, V.A. (1987) *Cranio-facial Growth during Adolesence*. Centre for Human Growth and Development, Ann Arbor, Michigan.

Enlow, D.H. (1982) *Handbook of Facial Growth*, 2nd ed. W.B. Saunders, Philadelphia.

Goose, D.H. & Appleton, J. (1982) *Human Dento-Facial growth*. Pergamon, Oxford.

Houston, W.J.B. (1979) The current status of facial growth prediction. *British Journal of Orthodontics*, **6**, 11.

Moyers, R.E., Van Der Linden, F.P.G.M., Riolo, M.L., McNamara, J.A. Jr (1976) *Standards of Human Occlusal Development*. University of Ann Arbor, Michigan.

Sinclair, D.C. (1982) *Human Growth after Birth*, 4th ed. Oxford Medical Publications.

Tanner, J.M. (1988) *Foetus into Man*. Open Books Ltd, Wells.

Woodside, D.G. & Linder-Aronson, S. (1979) The channelization of upper and lower facial heights compared to population standards in males. *European Journal of Orthodontics*, **1**, 25.

Chapter 3   Mode of Action

The precise mode of action of functional appliances is not fully understood. Although certain basic principles are common to all appliances of the functional group, individual variation in design may influence the effect of a particular type of appliance.

There is a wide variety of functional appliances but they all have one thing in common, that is that they hold the mandible away from its normal resting position. Protagonists of particular appliances make claims for their design, often implying some special quality which is not found in other appliances. In reality each appliance is constructed from a number of components and each component serves a purpose. Knowledge of how appliances work, and the various effects that the components may have, will enable the clinician to choose the appliance which is most suitable for a particular malocclusion, or indeed make modifications to an appliance in order to obtain the best effect. An excellent review of the action of the components of appliances is given by Vig & Vig (1986). In essence, functional appliances can have three broad methods of action which, although described separately, are closely interrelated.

1 Tipping movements

Tipping movements occur in both the labial and buccal teeth. Such movements are the same as those which can be carried out with conventional appliances and occur either as a result of contact between the appliance and the teeth, or due to altered muscle pressure induced by the appliance.

2 Eruption guidance

This is the mechanism whereby the vertical development of any group of teeth can be enhanced, inhibited, or redirected and thus assist in alteration of occlusal relationships. It is similar to the effect of a bite plane or molar capping of a conventional removable appliance.

3 Mandibular reposturing

This is the aspect of functional appliances which distinguishes them from any other appliance. The appliances are constructed with the mandible held in a postured position, and with the teeth out of occlusion; in the Class II case the mandible is held in a forward posture. The facial musculature is in a stretched position, and it is thought that, either as a result of reflex activity, or the elastic properties of the stretched muscles, forces are generated which can alter the bony development of the maxilla and mandible. The effect of occlusal separation is also considered to have an influence on the skeletal development. The removal of the influence of the occlusion of the lower incisors and of the intercuspation of the posterior teeth is said to permit full expression of mandibular growth. This change in mandibular and maxillary growth is called by some an 'orthopaedic' effect, and can only take place during periods of active growth. The majority of research papers on functional appliance treatment concentrate on this effect.

Importance of growth

Some advocate the use of functional appliances in the adult. Of the types of tooth movement outlined above tipping movements can take place at any age. A functional appliance in an adult can produce these dento-alveolar changes. Eruption guidance will be very limited and unpredictable in the non-growing patient, whilst the so-called orthopaedic effect from mandibular reposturing will be absent in the adult.

The authors consider that the dento-alveolar changes in the adult are achieved more easily with conventional appliance systems. McNamara (1984) reports three cases of adults treated with functional appliances and noted that the malocclusion present at the beginning of treatment was still present to a large degree at the end of treatment.

With conventional appliances growth may be desirable but when using functional appliances growth is essential (Fig. 3.1). Whilst success can be achieved in some cases in the pre- or postpubertal growth period the optimum time should include the period of maximum growth velocity (Fig. 3.2). However, it cannot be assumed that treatment by means of functional appliances will enhance growth of the jaws.

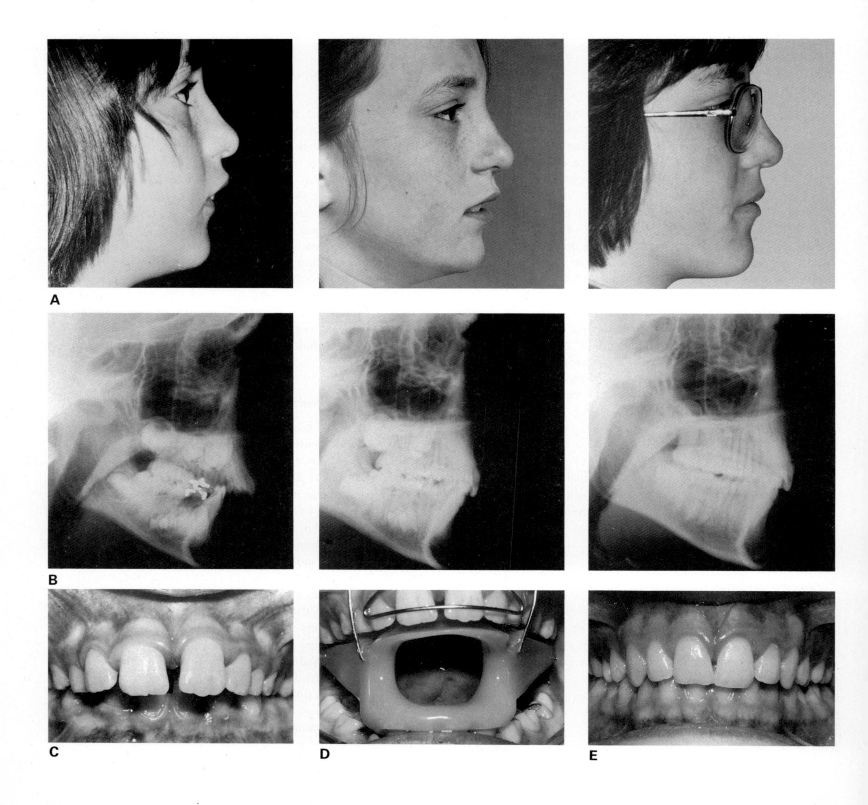

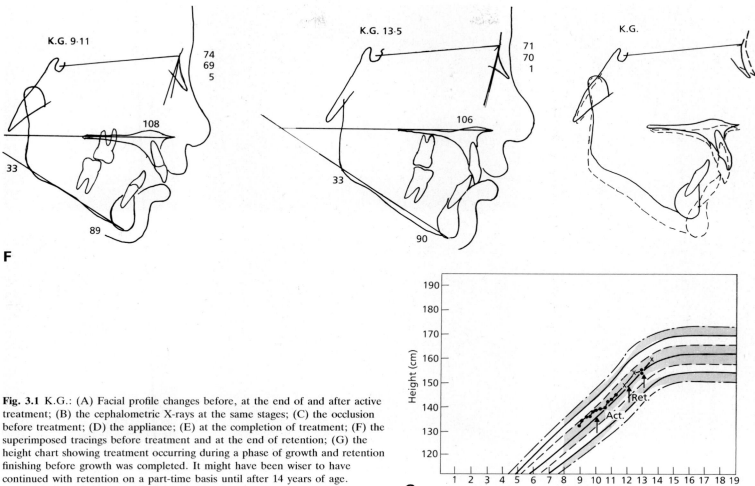

Fig. 3.1 K.G.: (A) Facial profile changes before, at the end of and after active treatment; (B) the cephalometric X-rays at the same stages; (C) the occlusion before treatment; (D) the appliance; (E) at the completion of treatment; (F) the superimposed tracings before treatment and at the end of retention; (G) the height chart showing treatment occurring during a phase of growth and retention finishing before growth was completed. It might have been wiser to have continued with retention on a part-time basis until after 14 years of age. Nevertheless the result in this case was stable.

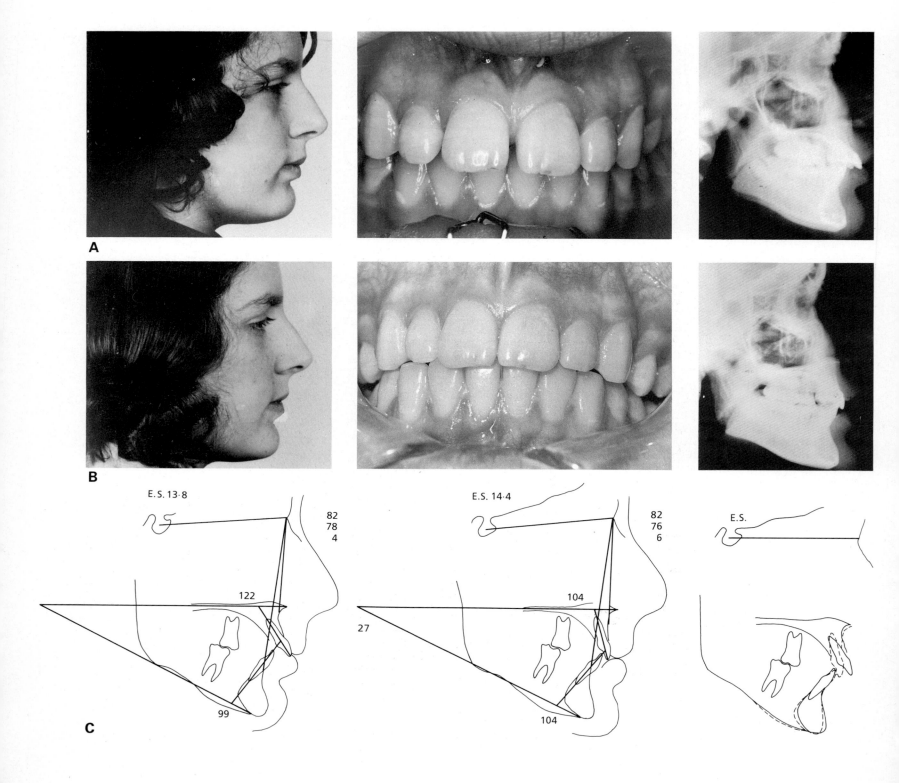

E.S. 13·8

82
78
4

122

99

E.S. 14·4

82
76
6

104

27

104

E.S.

A

B

C

Tipping movements

There are two effects of tipping movement to consider: the labio-lingual change that occurs in the incisor region, and the bucco-lingual change that takes place in the molar and pre-molar region.

Upper incisors

Retroclination is achieved by wire contact on the labial surface of the incisors with relief of contact on the palatal aspect. This treatment will require appropriate incisor spacing and may be indicated to a limited extent in the management of certain Class II division 1 cases.

Palatal retraction of upper incisors must be carefully controlled and is only permissible when the upper incisors are proclined. Retroclination should not move the teeth beyond the ideal inclination, otherwise it is not possible to establish a satisfactory inter-incisal angle at the end of treatment and the appearance may be poor. Proclination of the upper incisors is achieved by lingual contact of either acrylic or wire. This can be aided by muscle displacement on the labial aspect of the teeth with acrylic pads. This is a tooth movement often required in Class III cases.

Lower incisors

Lingual tipping is achieved by wire contact on the labial surface of the incisors with appropriate relief of contact on the lingual side. This tipping movement will require incisor spacing and is only indicated in Class III cases.

Proclination can be achieved by the contact of wire or acrylic on the lingual aspect of the teeth. This movement can be aided by muscle relief on the labial side by means of suitable shields or lip bumpers. Such a tooth movement is required in only a small

Fig. 3.2 (*facing page*) E.S.: (A) The records before the start of treatment; (B) the records at the end of active treatment. These show a pleasing change in the incisor relationship on the clinical photograph and the lateral skull X-ray. The facial profile however shows little change. (C) Tracings from the lateral skull X-rays show that the improvement in incisor relationship has been achieved entirely by dento-alveolar tooth movements. There has been some slight clockwise rotation of the mandible due to reduction in overbite. The patient commenced treatment after she had completed most of her growth.

proportion of cases and usually appliance design is aimed at preventing this in Class II cases, although it may be encouraged in Class II division 2 cases.

In the majority of malocclusions active lower incisor pro-clination is undesirable. Because of the well-known tendency of functional appliances to procline lower incisors, present-day designs usually attempt to minimize this movement. This can be achieved by reducing contact on the lingual aspect and providing a restraining influence on the labial aspect of the lower incisors.

Upper posterior teeth

In the upper arch, buccal tooth movement will occur as a result of pressure from the appliance on the palatal aspect; often active components such as springs or screws are used. Buccal movement can also be achieved by altering muscle balance. Buccal acrylic or wire shields hold the cheeks away from the teeth while the tongue pressure remains on the palatal side.

An increase in the intermolar width can occur without active components or change in muscle balance; this may be due to normal growth coupled with the change in occlusal relationship from Class II to Class I. Such a phenomenon is observed when using the activator which does not incorporate active components or buccal shields.

Palatal movement of upper posterior teeth is rarely required and can only be achieved by full-time appliance wear incorporating active components such as open screws.

Lower posterior teeth

Deliberate buccal movement can be achieved by altering muscle balance with buccal shields, allowing the effect of tongue pressure to be unrestricted. For these forces to be effective, occlusal interference from the upper teeth must be removed and this occurs with most functional appliances as a result of mandibular posturing. On the rare occasions when lingual movement of lower posterior teeth is required this is best carried out by fixed appliances.

Inter-arch bucco-lingual movement

In planning treatment the dento-alveolar changes that are required need careful attention when considering appliance design. The amount of expansion should only be sufficient to achieve or maintain a satisfactory intercuspation. In a growing patient some of the expansion occurs physiologically provided that the appliance design permits this. Active expansion should be sufficient only to allow for the correction of crossbites and should not be carried out in an attempt to relieve crowding. It is important to avoid an increase in lower intercanine width as this produces an unstable position which will almost inevitably relapse following treatment, causing lower incisor crowding.

Eruption guidance

During the process of normal facial growth the face grows downwards and forwards away from the base of the skull, and there is an increase in the distance between the upper and lower dental bases, which is filled by the developing alveolar processes. Functional appliances, especially the acrylic-based varieties, can be so designed as to modify this eruptive process. Selective inhibition of vertical development of groups of teeth can assist in the correction of a malocclusion.

Labial segments

Inhibition of vertical development of the labial segments is commonly seen in the well-documented bite plane effect of a conventional upper removable appliance (Cousins *et al*. 1969). An anterior bite plane restrains the vertical development of the lower incisors, whilst the removal of occlusal forces allows enhanced vertical development of both the upper and lower posterior teeth. The most common indication for this movement is where overbite reduction is required by flattening of the lower occlusal plane.

Control of the lower incisor vertical development is most easily achieved by the acrylic-based appliances. These can provide acrylic capping which covers the incisal edges, and the design of the appliances allows the lower posterior teeth to develop vertically. To a limited extent the more flexible wire-based appliances can also achieve this by contact of lingual wires on the lower incisors. Such wires, in addition to restricting vertical development, tend to cause proclination of the lower incisors.

It is unusual to achieve intrusion of the upper incisors by capping them and by leaving the molars out of contact with the appliance. This would allow downward and forward eruption of the upper posterior teeth which is undesirable in a Class II case.

Posterior teeth

Serial cephalometric studies have revealed that the eruption of both maxillary and mandibular posterior teeth is accompanied by mesial movement. By restricting either of these normal eruption patterns during treatment a change in the molar relationship can be obtained (Fig. 3.3). For Class II correction this is brought about by allowing free development of the lower posterior teeth while preventing any such movement in the upper. Conversely in Class III correction upwards and forwards development of the

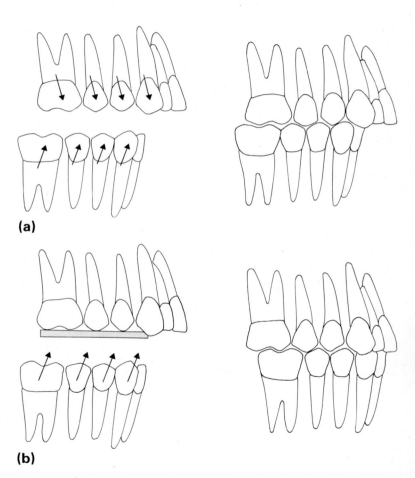

(a)

(b)

Fig. 3.3 (a) The development of an untreated Class II malocclusion. The uninhibited forward movement of both upper and lower posterior teeth maintains the Class II relationship. (b) With an occlusal shelf the maxillary posterior teeth are inhibited. Vertical and forward development of the lower posterior teeth allows a change to a Class I molar relationship.

lower posterior teeth is restrained whilst vertical development of the upper posterior teeth is permitted. In a Class II case the occlusal plane is tilted upwards at the back and in a Class III case the occlusal plane is tilted downwards at the back. For high angle cases and anterior openbite cases both the upper and lower posterior teeth are prevented from erupting whilst the anteriors are free to do so. This differential control was first described by Harvold and is particularly associated with his version of the activator with its plain occlusal shelves in the buccal region.

In the Andresen appliance, complex trimming of the acrylic in the buccal segments is required to give facets which are designed to encourage specific direction of the eruptive movements of the upper and lower posterior teeth. In the upper arch buccal movement is encouraged in Class II treatment by selective trimming of the acrylic to contact the mesial and palatal aspect of the posterior teeth. This produces a channel which directs the teeth occlusally, distally and buccally. The converse is advocated in the lower arch. More recent experience seems to indicate that such trimming is not necessary.

Mandibular reposturing — the orthopaedic effect

Some consider that functional appliances act solely by simple mechanical means: in other words the appliance forms a method of applying a force between the arches, in the same way that elastic traction can in fixed appliance treatment. The muscular action simply replaces the pull or traction of the elastics. The opposing view is that the appliances, by providing a new muscular and functional environment of the facial bones, encourage additional growth of either the mandible or the maxilla, as appropriate.

There is evidence to suggest that the simple mechanical theory is not always sufficient to account for all the changes that take place in patients who are successfully treated with functional appliances (Fig. 3.4). The effects of functional appliances on the maxilla and mandible differ and will be considered separately.

The maxilla

In the treatment of Class II malocclusions, the normal forward and downward growth pattern of the maxilla is restrained due to the action of the appliance, with both sutural lowering of the maxilla and growth in height of the alveolar process being in-hibited (Fig. 3.5). It is possible that the lip posture may also have an influence on the maxillary development. With functional appliances in position, the mandible is usually held so that it is possible for the lower lip to be brought in front of the upper incisors, this action aiding the restriction of maxillary dento-alveolar growth. The growth restriction observed is similar to that seen when headgear forces are used for long periods of time in the treatment of Class II malocclusions.

In the management of Class III cases it is argued that functional appliances can stimulate maxillary forward growth, particularly by surface deposition of bone. Appliances to treat Class III occlusions usually incorporate labial shields or wires to hold the upper lip away from the maxillary alveolar process (Fig. 3.6). Indeed, advocates of certain appliances recommend stretching of the lips. There is little evidence, either clinical or from animal research, to support this view.

The mandible

The mandible may be affected in three ways: the appliance makes the mandible grow longer, the rate of growth of the mandible may be increased, or the direction of growth may be improved.

TOTAL GROWTH

Protagonists claim that growth of the mandible, particularly at the condyle, is increased by functional appliances. This is said to be through stimulation of the condylar cartilage in response to the distraction of the head of the condyle from the fossa. The mandible responds, according to the functional matrix theory of Moss (1968), by the addition of extra bone to compensate for its new position. In clinical practice, cases are seen where it might appear that the mandible has grown during treatment, but this may be no greater than the amount of growth that would have taken place without treatment. The restriction of the growth of the maxilla and other factors are often sufficient to correct the Class II relationship. Research so far suggests that, on average, 1 mm of additional bone growth of the mandible can be expected. This on its own does not wholly account for the changes frequently seen in clinical practice. However, it must be borne in mind that this figure represents the mean for experimental groups: the range is probably large, and may explain why certain cases appear to show a response much greater than this amount (Fig. 3.7).

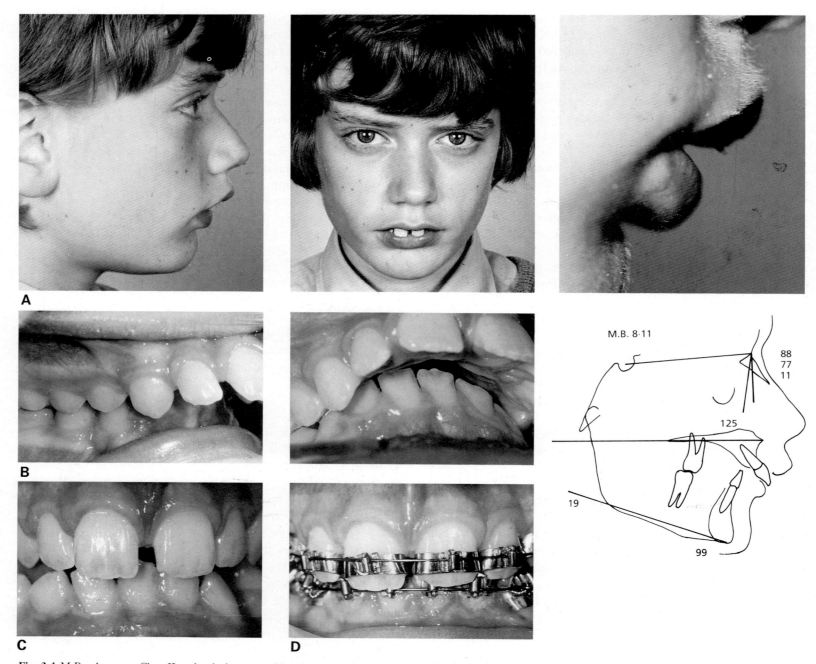

Fig. 3.4 M.B.: A severe Class II malocclusion treated by a combination of functional appliances, premolar extractions and fixed appliance. (A) The initial facial appearance; (B) the initial occlusion with an overjet of 18 mm; (C) overjet reduction at the end of the activator stage of treatment; (D) fixed appliance for final correction; (E) final facial appearance; (F) the occlusion 3 years out of retention.

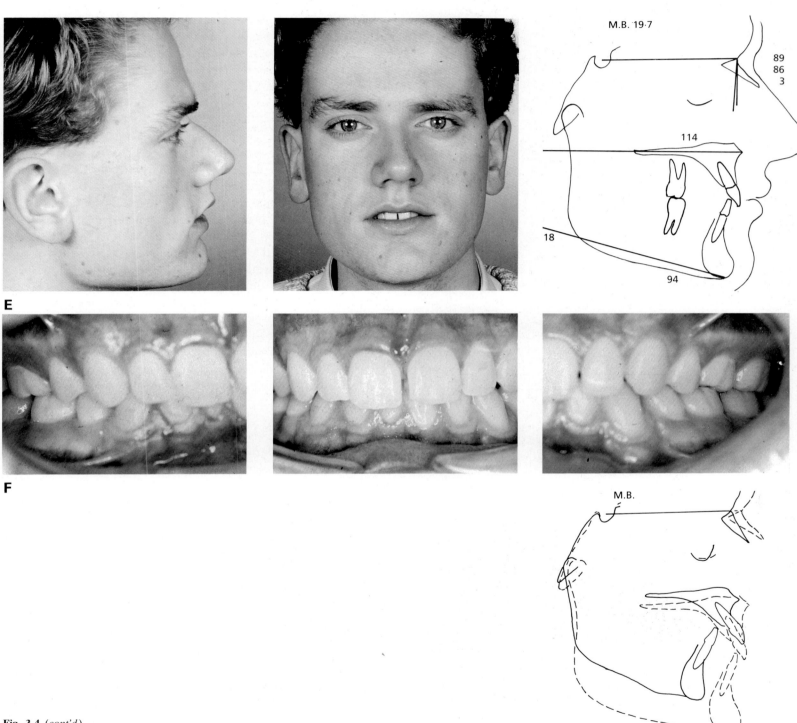

Fig. 3.4 (*cont'd*)

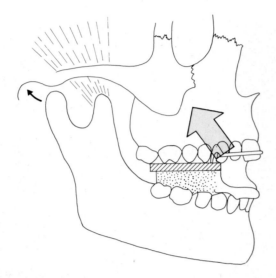

Fig. 3.5 Inhibition of maxillary development may take place at both sutural and alveolar sites.

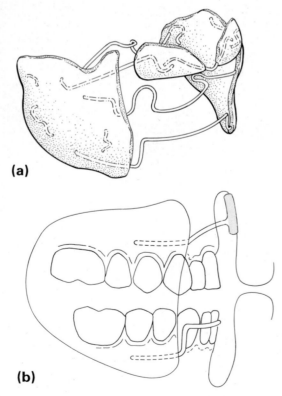

(a)

(b)

Fig. 3.6 (a) FR3 with maxillary labial pads; (b) position of upper labial pad.

In the management of Class III occlusions, there is no scientific evidence for the restriction of mandibular growth, whether by the use of extra oral forces, chin caps or functional appliances. This is in contrast with Class II cases where the number of successfully treated cases is large (Fig. 3.8).

DIRECTION OF GROWTH

Normal mandibular growth of the facial skeleton is downwards and forwards, with the dento-alveolar processes developing to maintain a constant freeway space. According to Björk there is considerable individual variation in the behaviour of the mandible during this growth process. Some mandibles appear to rotate backwards, which is generally unfavourable, especially in the treatment of Class II cases. Fortunately, in the majority of subjects, the mandible rotates forwards during growth.

The influence of functional appliances on this process is controversial. Most workers have suggested that the bite plane effect tends to produce backward rotation. Studies by Luder (1983) have suggested that the direction of growth can be altered to a more favourable forward rotation by influencing the direction of growth at the condyle (Fig. 3.9). In normal clinical practice, such changes are impossible to detect during treatment.

RATE OF GROWTH

It is possible that, during the period of treatment, the growth of the mandible is accelerated. This can occur with or without an increase in the final length of the mandible. Several workers have found that the rate of growth is enhanced during treatment. This is probably beneficial in aiding correction of the incisor and buccal segment relationship. Once a Class I relationship is established the lips can come into a new position controlling the upper labial segment, and the relative rate of growth of the mandible reduces so that the final growth of the maxilla and mandible is in harmony (Fig. 3.10).

GLENOID FOSSA

It is postulated that the continued forward position of the condyle causes resorption of the anterior border of the glenoid fossa, and that remodelling of this allows further forward positioning of the mandible (Fig. 3.11). This gives a new position of the mandible.

Animal experimentation by Hinton & McNamara (1984) and clinical papers by Birkbebaek, Melsen & Terp (1984) have indicated that this is a possibility but the ability to identify the fossa accurately on radiographs is such that any small changes would be difficult to demonstrate.

MUSCULAR ACTION

Opinions differ greatly on the effect of functional appliances on the muscles of mastication or the facial muscles. The simplest explanation of the action of muscle forces is that in response to the mandibular displacement caused by the appliance, the elastic stretch of the muscles acts in the same way as intermaxillary elastic traction. This applies a Class II or Class III correction force between the maxilla and mandible. Animal experiments by Yemm (1975) elegantly show that the forces involved in enforced jaw opening, in the rat at least, are related principally to elastic stretch (Fig. 3.12).

The alternative view is that myotactic reflexes are brought into play by the action of the appliance and the muscles are stimulated to produce an isometric contraction. The muscles are re-educated to accept the mandible in its new postural position, and growth of the maxilla and mandible reflects this.

The circum-oral musculature may be influential in applying forces to the dento-alveolar structures. The positioning of the mandible by the appliance frequently puts the lower lip in a new position relative to the upper incisors. This has two effects. Firstly, it removes the lower lip from below and behind the upper incisors, and any forward development of the mandible and lower lip is not then transferred to the palatal aspect of the upper incisors. Secondly, the lower lip, when in front of the upper incisors, offers a restraining force on the incisors and possibly also on the development of the maxilla. The patient will frequently make a conscious effort to achieve a lip seal, which in turn increases the force on the upper arch (Fig. 3.13).

In considering the two theories of muscular action with functional appliances, it is probable that both types of action occur to a greater or lesser extent, and are dependent upon the type of appliance used. The more flexible appliances, which on the whole have minimum opening and allow for mandibular movement, are most likely to evoke a neuro-muscular response with isometric muscle contraction being responsible for providing the force. The more rigid appliances, particularly those which have a considerable mandibular opening, are more likely to act by passive stretch of the muscles (Woodside et al., 1973).

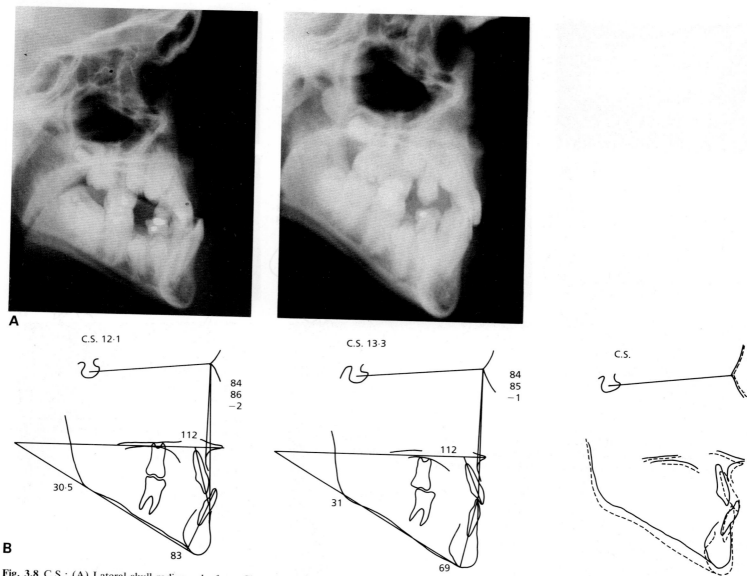

Fig. 3.8 C.S.: (A) Lateral skull radiographs for a Class III malocclusion treated with an activator. Superficial inspection of these radiographs might lead the clinician to suppose that there has been a significant change in the underlying skeletal pattern as a result of treatment. (B) The tracings and superimposition taken from these radiographs show that the favourable occlusal change has been brought about entirely by dento-alveolar tooth movement and the elimination of mandibular displacement. The underlying skeletal pattern remains the same.

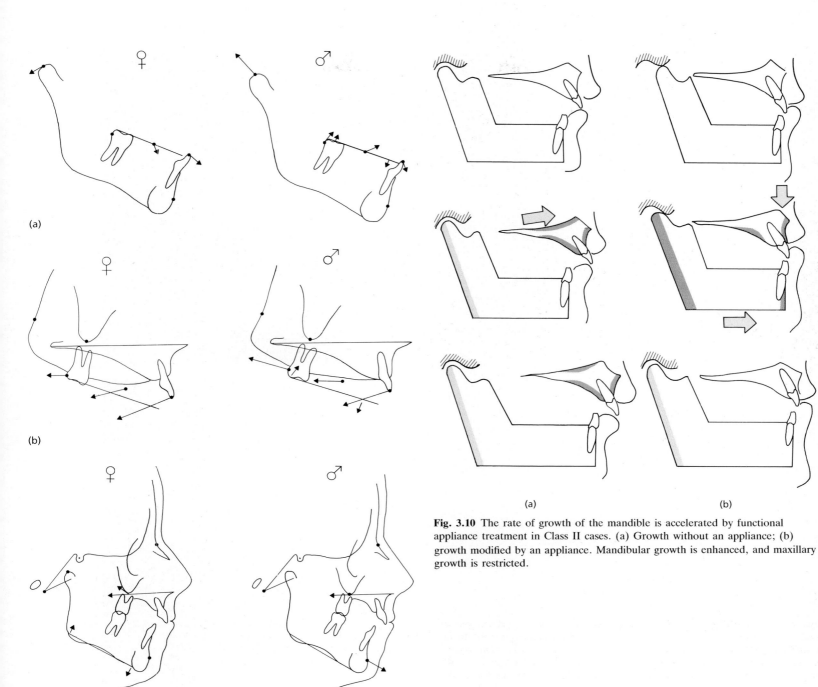

Fig. 3.10 The rate of growth of the mandible is accelerated by functional appliance treatment in Class II cases. (a) Growth without an appliance; (b) growth modified by an appliance. Mandibular growth is enhanced, and maxillary growth is restricted.

Fig. 3.9 The comparison between males and females treated with functional appliances (redrawn after Luder 1983). The size of the arrows represents 10 times the measured changes: (a) Effect on the mandible; (b) effect on the maxilla; (c) overall effect.

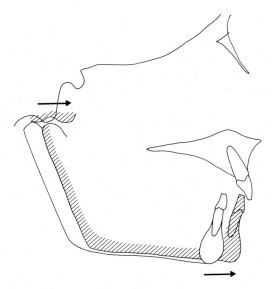

Fig. 3.11 Remodelling of the glenoid fossa permits forward translation of the mandible.

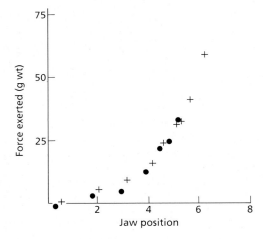

Fig. 3.12 The graph shows the force applied to displace a rat's mandible plotted against the amount of opening. The dots represent the readings taken whilst the animal was lightly anaesthetized and the crosses the readings taken shortly after the rat was sacrificed. This suggests that muscle elasticity and gravity are mostly responsible for the control of the mandibular rest position (after Yemm 1975).

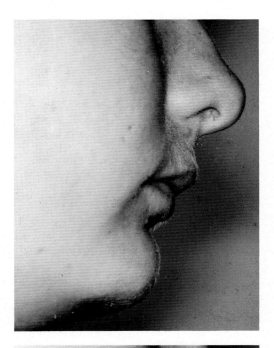

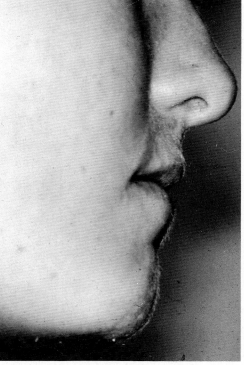

Fig. 3.13 The effect of lip seal with and without an activator.

References

Birkbebaek, L., Melsen, B. & Terp, S. (1984) A laminographic study of the temporo-mandibular joint following activator treatment. *European Journal of Orthodontics*, **6**, 257.

Cousins, A.J.P., Brown, W.A.B. & Harkness, E.M. (1969) An investigation into the effect of the maxillary bite plate on the height of the lower incisor teeth. *Transactions of the British Society for the Study of Orthodontics*, 105.

Hinton, R.J. & McNamara, J.A. Jr (1984) Temple bone adaptations in Rhesus monkeys. *European Journal of Orthodontics*, **6**, 155.

Luder, H.V. (1983) The effect of activator treatment. *European Journal of Orthodontics*, **5**, 259.

McNamara, J.A. Jr (1984) Dentofacial adaptations in adult patients following functional regulator therapy. *American Journal of Orthodontics*, **85**, 57.

Moss, M.L. (1968) The primacy of functional matrix in orofacial growth. *Dental Practitioner*, **19**, 65.

Vig, P.S. & Vig, K.W. (1986) Hybrid appliances, a component approach to dento-facial orthopaedics. *American Journal of Orthodontics*, **90**, 273.

Woodside, D.G., Reed, R.T., Doucet, J.D. & Thompson, G.W. (1973) Some effects of activator treatment on the mandible and midface. *Transactions of the European Orthodontic Society*, 443.

Yemm, R. (1975) The mandibular rest position. *Journal of the South African Dental Association*, **30**, 203.

Further reading

Björk, A. & Skieller, V. (1983) Normal and abnormal growth of mandible. A synthesis of longitudinal cephalometric implant studies over a period of 25 years. *European Journal of Orthodontics*, **5**, 1.

Harvold, D.E. & Vargevik, K. (1971) The morphogenetic response to the activator. *American Journal of Orthodontics*, **60**, 478.

McNamara, J.A. Jr (1980) Functional determinants of craniofacial size and shape. *European Journal of Orthodontics*, **2**, 131.

Williams, S. & Melsen, B. (1982) The interplay between sagittal and vertical growth factors. *American Journal of Orthodontics*, **81**, 327.

Yemm, R. & Nordstrom, S.H. (1974) Forces developed by tissue elasticity as a determinant of mandibular resting posture in the rat. *Archives Oral Biology*, **19**, 347.

Chapter 4   Cephalometry

Cephalometric assessment

Cephalometric radiographs are used extensively in orthodontics both in the assessment of malocclusion and the management of treatment. Where treatment with the active plate type of removable appliance is properly confined to cases with near-normal skeletal relationships it is possible to undertake this without assistance from cephalometry. However, where functional or fixed appliances are to be used the cephalometric radiograph is of great importance in the accurate diagnosis and successful execution of treatment. In general, cephalometry is required to fulfill one or more of the following purposes:

1 As an aid to assessment of the skeletal pattern of the malocclusion, by determining the relationship of the dental bases to each other (antero-posterior and vertical) and to the cranial base.

2 The prediction of the likely direction and effect of future cranio-facial growth.

3 As a method of monitoring treatment progress and growth changes.

4 To acquire data from which retrospective and prospective research studies of groups of patients can be made.

In any assessment it must be remembered that a cephalometric radiograph is a magnified two-dimensional image of a three-dimensional object. This means that where the images of bilateral structures appear on the film they will have been magnified by unequal amounts. Furthermore, distances between points will be magnified by unequal amounts unless all the points lie at the same distance from the film. Fortunately most of the points which are used in lateral cephalometry are found on single structures which lie in or are close to the mid-sagittal plane of the head.

Analysis of the cephalometric film is carried out using a number of standard anatomical landmarks which can be easily and reproducibly identified on the lateral projection. Usually tracings are made to enable angular and linear measurements to be recorded and analysed. Most analyses compare data from the individual with mean values for the population from which the patient has been drawn. In making such comparisons, angular measurements and linear measurements expressed as ratios are more valuable, as these avoid problems arising from changes in the size of the facial skeleton of the growing child. Some clinicians use these norms as aims for treatment, attempting to correct an individual patient to a set of standard cephalometric values. Whilst such an aim may be realistic for milder malocclusions the degree to which facial shape can be changed by treatment is such that in severe malocclusion the cephalometric assessment can only offer guidance as to the most appropriate line of treatment.

Some clinicians, and more recently certain commercial organizations, believe that they can make a clinically useful prediction of growth changes to aid treatment planning. These are made by adding average increments of growth to data from the patient's radiograph. Unfortunately there is no way in which individual variation can be adequately catered for when using a single radiograph even if the average increments have been derived from an appropriate population (same race, same sex, same facial type and same age).

Commonly used analyses

Eastman analysis

This is the most frequently used analysis in the United Kingdom and is derived from the work of Downs & Reidel (Brown 1981). It employs the following points and planes (Fig. 4.1):

1 Sella—the centre of the sella turcica.

2 Nasion—the junction of the nasal bone and the frontal bone.

3 A-point—the greatest concavity on the alveolar labial plate of the maxillary bone in the midline.

4 B-point—the greatest labial concavity of the mandibular alveolus in the midline.

5 The maxillary plane—from the anterior to posterior nasal spine.

6 Menton—the lowest point of the mandibular symphysis.

7 Gonion—the most inferior and posterior point at the angle of the mandible.

8 The mandibular plane—a line passing through menton and gonion generally taken to represent the lower border of the mandible.

9 The upper incisor angulation to the maxillary plane.

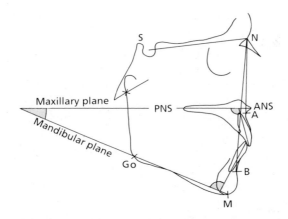

Fig. 4.1 Standard cephalometric points and planes (after Houston): A = A-point; B = B-point; S = sella; N = nasion; Go = gonion; M = menton; Ar = articulare; ANS = anterior nasal spine; PNS = posterior nasal spine.

10 The lower incisor angulation to the mandibular plane.

11 The ratio of the upper to lower facial height expressed as a percentage of the total face height. The upper facial height is from nasion to anterior nasal spine: the lower facial height from anterior nasal spine to menton.

The assessment of skeletal Class (sagittal relationship of the jaws) is achieved by looking at the angles between the A-point, nasion and B-point (the ANB angle). The range of the ANB angle in a Class 1 case is 2−4 degrees. Below this, that is less than 2 degrees, indicates a Class 3 pattern. A value greater than 4 degrees demonstrates a Class 2 jaw relationship (Fig. 4.2). Unfortunately the reliability of the ANB angle as a measure of skeletal discrepancy is affected by the relative protrusion, or retrusion, of the lower face with respect to the cranial base. This is reflected in the value of the SNA angle. It is generally assumed that the values given above for the ANB angle are only correct for an SNA angle of 81 degrees. Where the facial shape is such that SNA is significantly above or below this value, correction must be made to the value of ANB. Conventionally 1 degree is added to ANB for each 3 degrees above the average SNA of 81 degrees, and 1 degree subtracted from ANB norms for each 3 degrees below the average SNA (Fig. 4.3). This method provides the simplest radiographic assessment of skeletal pattern. It also gives an indication of the relative contribution made by the protrusion or retrusion of maxilla and mandible to the cranium.

Some problems are associated with the interpretation of this

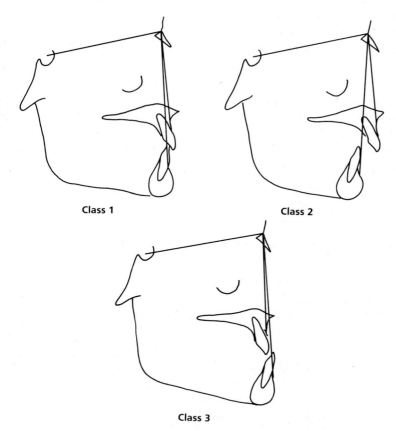

Fig. 4.2 Class 1, Class 2 and Class 3 skeletal patterns as defined by the ANB angle.

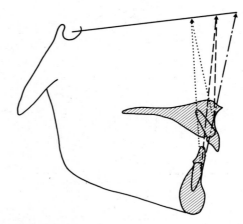

Fig. 4.3 Variation in the position of the nasion can influence the value of the ANB angle.

analysis. The labial plate varies in thickness and the A-point changes its position during tipping of incisors. Another difficulty arises when the position of the sella is low and an abnormally small value of SNA and SNB results: for this type of facial form, correction of the ANB angle described above is inappropriate.

The maxillary–mandibular planes angle, the angulation of the upper incisors to the maxillary plane, and of the lower incisors to the mandibular plane, are highly relevant for assessment and treatment planning for the patient.

The lower facial height is expressed as a percentage of total facial height and this overcomes the problem of individual variation in size. This percentage (53% to 55%) normally remains fairly constant throughout facial development and so a change during treatment usually indicates a treatment effect (Fig. 4.4).

Harvold analysis

This analysis uses linear measurements and attempts to take account of the effect of the lower face height on the sagittal relationship of the jaws. For example, consider a patient with an ideal relationship of his jaws both to each other and to the cranial base. If for some reason the patient's lower face height increased, the mandible would become posteriorly positioned as it hinged open, and a skeletal 2 dental base relationship would develop. If on the other hand the lower face height reduced, the mandible

would rotate upwards and forwards and a skeletal 3 relationship would develop. This is a simplification to illustrate the underlying principle. In reality such changes take place in a growing patient where vertical changes in face height may to a greater or lesser extent be offset by differences in horizontal growth of the mandible and maxilla. In the Harvold analysis individual variation is partially overcome by taking both maxillary and mandibular measurements from the same point. The distance from a point on the glenoid fossa to the front of the maxillary plane at the anterior nasal spine is designated the maxillary unit length (Tables 4.1 and 4.2) and that from the same glenoid point to the chin point, the mandibular unit length (Fig. 4.5; Tables 4.3 and 4.4). The difference between these two dimensions forms the assessment of the skeletal pattern in the sagittal plane (Table 4.5). When growth is completed a difference in the two lengths of between 22 to 27 mm defines skeletal Class 1, less than this Class 2, and more than this Class 3, and the relative changes of arch length during the treatment indicate an improvement in the skeletal relationship due either to mandibular lengthening or restriction of maxillary growth.

One of the problems encountered when using this assessment is the difficulty in defining the head of the condyle. Articulare is used by some clinicians but does not demonstrate the full length of the mandible to which published data refer. However, the analysis has the advantage of drawing the clinician's attention to

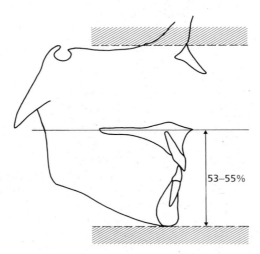

Fig. 4.4 The lower facial height as a percentage of total facial height (53–55%) tends to remain constant for the untreated individual. Changes in this value are usually attributed to treatment.

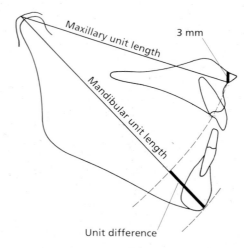

Fig. 4.5 The Harvold analysis. (The maxillary unit length is taken to the bottom of a line drawn at right angles to the maxillary plane through the anterior nasal spine at a point where it is 3 mm thick.)

increase in the maxillary–mandibular planes angle and an increase in lower facial height. In the absence of treatment the maxillary–mandibular planes angle reduces with growth. A geometric result of this increase in face height is that the B-point not only goes downwards but backwards, increasing the ANB angle slightly (Fig. 4.11). It should be borne in mind that in due time the lower border of the mandible will remodel and thus the maxillary–mandibular planes angle will return to near its original value even though the face height remains increased. This change is sometimes referred to as a clockwise rotation of the mandible (on the assumption that the patient is viewed with the head facing to the right).

Lower incisor angulation

Most orthodontic practice in the UK is based on the premise that the labial position of the lower incisor tip should not be altered during treatment (Mills 1966). Simple proclination of lower incisors is unlikely to be stable. Treatment should therefore be aimed at keeping the lower incisor position constant. Functional appliances, by virtue of their construction, tend to procline the lower incisors. Appliances should be constructed so as to minimize or avoid this unwanted tooth movement.

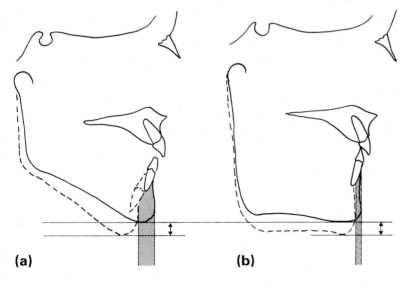

(a)   **(b)**

Fig. 4.11 The effect of an increase in face height during treatment: (a) A high MM angle case is more detrimental to the sagittal jaw relationship than (b) a low MM angle case.

Upper incisor angulation

The aim of treatment in a Class II division 1 case is to reduce the overjet, and produce a stable incisor occlusion, which is aesthetically pleasing. If overjet reduction is achieved with excessive incisor tipping, a satisfactory inter-incisal angle cannot be achieved. This can result in a lack of vertical stability leading to an increase in incisor overbite. Simple appliances, such as removable appliances, can only tip the incisors palatally. In cases with minimal skeletal discrepancy and proclined incisors, this may produce a good incisor occlusion. For more difficult cases most orthodontists use fixed appliances with the aim of restriction of the amount of incisor tipping which takes place during overjet reduction.

Functional appliances, when used in a growing patient, appear to achieve overjet reduction with less incisor tipping than the use of fixed appliances alone, provided there is no activation of the labial bow (Hawthorn 1987).

Summary

Cephalometric measurements must be used with caution. They must not be used as an arithmetical method of planning treatment, nor can they be used at our present state of knowledge to make claims that a certain form of treatment has stimulated mandibular growth. They are, however, the most important method available for measuring the changes that take place, and are a valuable source of data for clinical research.

Table 4.1 Maxillary unit length in males

Age (years)	Length (mm)	
	Mean value	Standard deviation
6	82	3.19
9	87	3.42
12	92	3.73
14	96	4.52
16	100	4.17

Table 4.2 Maxillary unit length in females

Age (years)	Length (mm) Mean value	Standard deviation
6	80	2.96
9	85	3.43
12	90	4.07
14	92	3.69
16	93	3.45

Table 4.3 Mandibular unit length in males

Age (years)	Length (mm) Mean value	Standard deviation
6	99	3.85
9	107	4.40
12	114	4.90
14	121	6.05
16	127	5.25

Table 4.4 Mandibular unit length in females

Age (years)	Length (mm) Mean value	Standard deviation
6	97	3.55
9	105	3.88
12	113	5.20
14	117	4.60
16	119	4.44

Table 4.5 Unit difference

Males		Females	
Age (years)	Length (mm) (mean value)	Age (years)	Length (mm) (mean value)
6	17	6	17
9	20	9	20
12	22	12	23
14	25	14	26
16	27	16	26

References

Björk, A., Skieller, V. (1983) Normal and abnormal growth of the mandible. *European Journal of Orthodontics*, **5**, 183.

Brown, M. (1981) Eight methods of analysing a cephalogram. *British Journal of Orthodontics*, **8**, 139.

Hawthorn, I.S. (1987) Apical root absorption incident to orthodontic treatment. MSc Report (abstract), *British Journal of Orthodontics*, **14**, 313.

Houston, W.J.B. & Lee, R.T. (1985) Accuracy of different methods of radiographic superimposition. *European Journal of Orthodontics*, **7**, 127.

Mills, J.R.E. (1966) The stability of the lower labial segment. *Dental Practice Dental Record*, **18**, 293.

Further reading

Björk, A.B. (1951) Significance of growth changes in facial pattern and their relationship to changes in occlusion. *Dental Record*, 197.

Harvold, E. (1974) *The activator in interceptive orthodontics*. Mosby, St Louis.

Horowitz, S.L. & Hixon, E.H. (1966) *The nature of orthodontic diagnosis*, Ch. 16. Mosby, St Louis.

Houston, W.J.B. (1982) *Orthodontic Diagnosis*, 3rd edn. J. Wright, Bristol.

Houston, W.J.B. (1983) The analysis of errors in orthodontic measurement. *American Journal of Orthodontics*, **83**, 382.

Houston, W.J.B. & Tulley, W.J. (1986) *A Textbook of Orthodontics*. J. Wright, Bristol.

Salzmann, J.A. (1974) *Orthodontics in Daily Practice*, Ch. 16, p. 197. Lippincott, Philadelphia.

Williams, P. (1986) Lower incisor position in treatment planning. *British Journal of Orthodontics*, **13**, 33.

Chapter 5   Case Selection and Management of Functional Appliances

Case selection

The traditional view that functional appliances are only suited to minimal Class II division 1 malocclusions with uncrowded lower arches has been largely discarded in recent years. Many workers now treat a much wider range of cases with functional appliances, albeit anticipating that many of them will require finishing with fixed appliances. Class II division 1 malocclusions form the majority of reported cases.

Social considerations

As discovered by Andresen, functional appliances may achieve their results with the minimum supervision and unlike fixed appliances can be worn safely for long periods without supervision. Unfortunately few cases are amenable for treatment by functional appliances alone, and it is therefore unwise to embark upon treatment in patients who are not available for regular attendance. Even in those cases where one might reasonably expect to achieve a result with functional appliances alone, the absence of regular appointments to encourage and motivate the patient may put the treatment in jeopardy. Hence patients who live far away from the surgery, or are attending boarding school, must have a very high level of self-motivation if satisfactory results are to be achieved.

Age

Almost all would agree that treatment can only be of clinical benefit to growing patients, the optimum time being between 10 years of age and the maximum pubertal growth spurt. There is no place for such appliance therapy in the adult patient.

Dental considerations

The chief contra-indication for functional appliance therapy is considerable local irregularity and rotation of incisors, especially the upper incisors. Crowding itself is not necessarily a contra-indication as this can be dealt with by extractions undertaken before, during or after functional appliance treatment. Only in uncrowded cases is it likely that a malocclusion can be treated to a satisfactory conclusion entirely with a functional appliance. In a small number of cases which demonstrate crowding but no significant anterior tooth irregularity or rotation treatment may be possible by a combination of extractions and functional appliances relying on spontaneous tooth movement to close any residual extraction space (Fig. 5.1). In most other cases, it is likely that a fixed appliance will be required to carry out detailed tooth alignment and space closure to complete treatment.

Skeletal considerations

In the antero-posterior plane, cases that are suitable for a functional appliance approach range from the moderate to the most severe skeletal 2. Mild Class II malocclusions can often be treated in a satisfactory fashion in the established permanent dentition by conventional means with or without extractions and the assistance of extra-oral forces. More severe skeletal 2 patterns will often benefit from a degree of modification during the growing phase by functional appliance techniques. This gives a better result than would have been the case if treatment had been based entirely upon conventional fixed appliance techniques. In some severe Class 2 cases the use of functional appliances can convert a case which potentially might require orthognathic surgery into one which can be managed by orthodontic means alone. Certain mild skeletal 3 cases can also be managed with a functional appliance (Loh & Kerr 1985).

CLASS II DIVISION 1 MALOCCLUSIONS

Mild Class II division 1 cases respond very well to functional appliance treatment especially if the arches are well-aligned. The advantage of the use of functional appliances in mild cases where pre-molar extractions are required must be questioned since such cases can be more effectively treated with the present-day sophisticated fixed appliances. By contrast more severe Class 2 cases may benefit from the use of functional appliances whether they are designated extraction or non-extraction. In non-

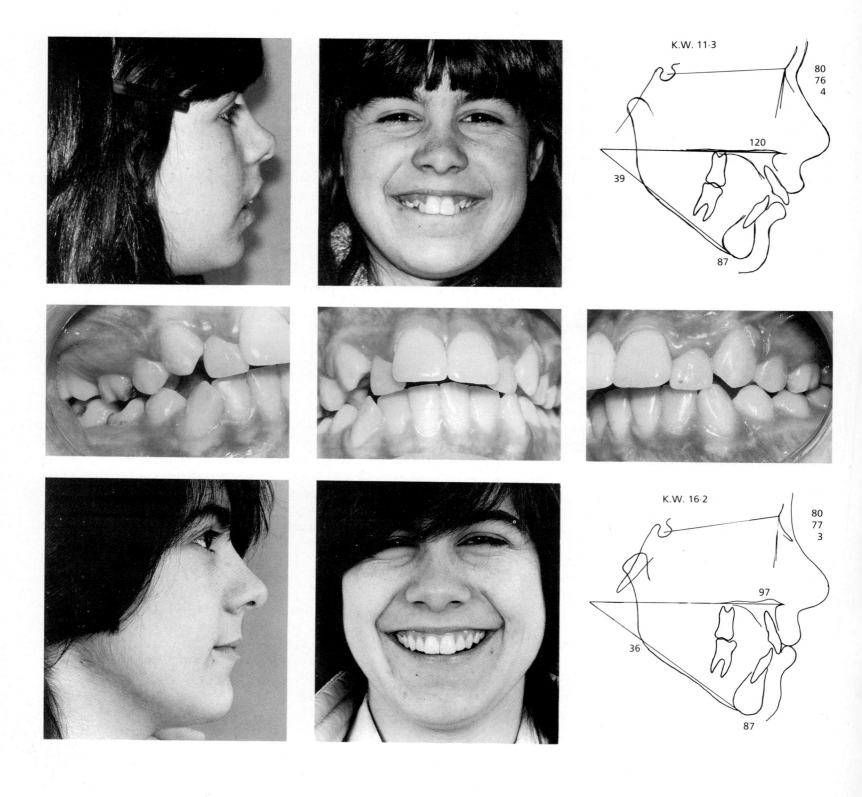

K.W. 11·3

80
76
4

120

39

87

K.W. 16·2

80
77
3

97

36

87

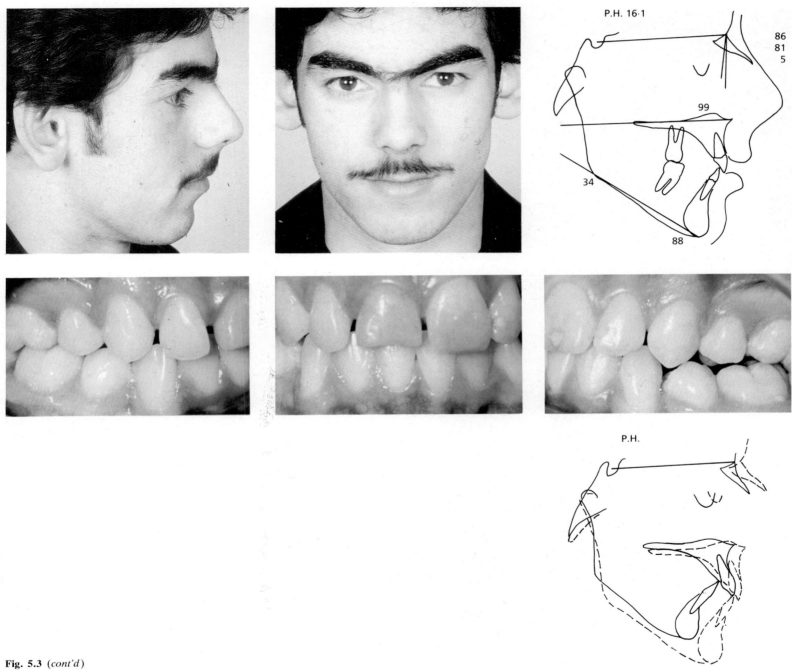

Fig. 5.3 (*cont'd*)

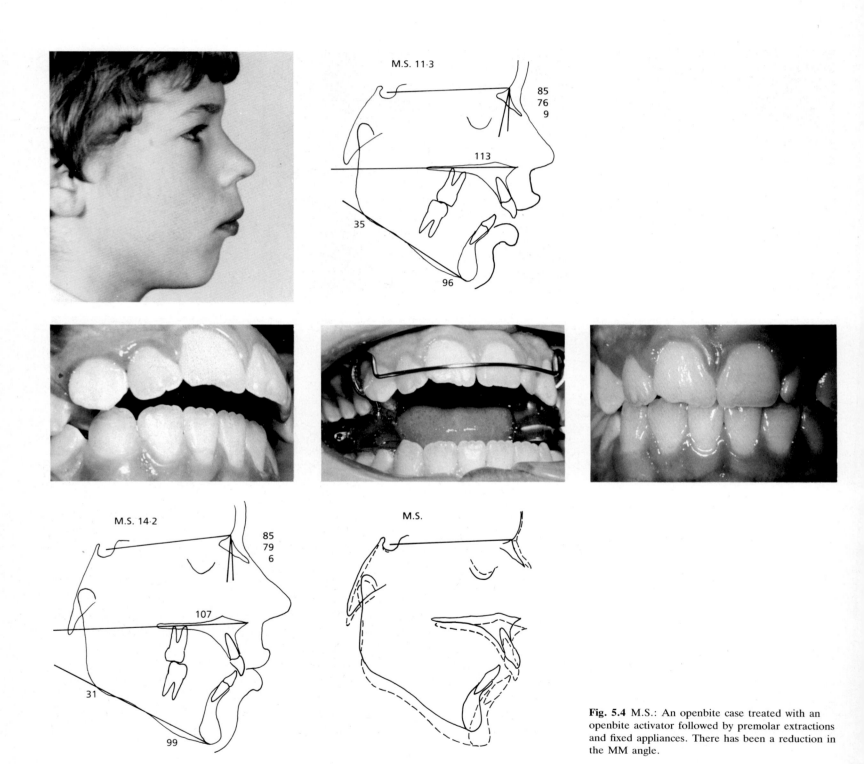

Fig. 5.4 M.S.: An openbite case treated with an openbite activator followed by premolar extractions and fixed appliances. There has been a reduction in the MM angle.

expected to grow in the immediate future. Local crowding or irregularity may contra-indicate such treatment or complicate the case. The place of functional appliance therapy in the treatment of other types of malocclusion is more controversial and much less well established.

Appliance management

This section gives general guidance on the management of functional appliances. For specific instructions concerning a particular appliance the reader is referred to the next chapter where each appliance is described in detail.

Patient motivation

As with all appliance systems it is essential for the orthodontist and patient to develop a rapport which will ensure satisfactory patient motivation and attention to details such as oral hygiene. Nowhere is this more evident than in the management of functional appliances.

Before commencing treatment it is necessary to give the patient and parents a very clear explanation of what is expected from the patient and what will be achieved by wearing the appliance. It must be made clear that the appliance is part of a total orthodontic treatment plan which may well need fixed appliances and headgear for completion of treatment. It is also wise to warn patients and parents that the extraction of permanent teeth is often necessary. Indeed before embarking upon treatment with a functional appliance it is essential to have seen the patient on his own to ensure that he is sufficiently well motivated to co-operate with this form of treatment. It is our view that a clear idea of potential patient co-operation cannot be obtained when this interview takes place in the presence of a parent.

Records

The normal clinical practice of having full records available before commencing orthodontic treatment should be followed. These records will include: models, photographs, appropriate radiographs (including cephalometric radiographs). In addition it is wise to record standing height in order to monitor growth changes.

Impression and occlusal registration

Working impressions are taken with particular reference to the appliance to be used. Care must be taken to ensure an adequately extended impression in the lingual and buccal sulcuses. It is often helpful to use wax on the periphery of the tray, and to 'muscle trim' this before taking the impression.

The working bite registration must be taken with care and must be related specifically to the appliance to be constructed but there is much variation in bite-taking techniques between different operators. Certain general principles apply. A clear imprint of the upper and lower dental arches must be made so that the laboratory can locate the models accurately. A thick wax bite wafer is required, and commercially produced ones are usually too thin (Fig. 5.7). For some appliances or malocclusions a wafer of up to 10 mm thickness may be required: for example a deep-bite Class II case, even with the bite taken with the incisors edge to edge, will have a separation of the posterior teeth of this order. It is wise to have a small stock of such wax bite wafers available. These are best made in soft-grade wax which in this thickness is sufficiently rigid, yet will readily take imprints of the teeth without distortion.

The first step in taking this record is to indent the upper teeth into the wax by firm pressure. To register the mandibular teeth in the postured position chosen, the patient's co-operation is necessary. The patient should hold a hand mirror and be instructed to move the lower incisors towards the chosen position. The patient should practice this once or twice before inserting the wax wafer. It may still require more than one attempt to achieve a satisfactory and consistent position. False registrations can be removed without heating the wax. The record can then be easily relocated accurately on the upper arch.

If the centre lines are not coincident at the start of treatment, the cause of the discrepancy should be ascertained. If a lateral displacing activity of the mandible is present then the working registration is taken so that the displacement is effectively eliminated. Where the centre line discrepancy is due to local dento-alveolar factors this is usually maintained in the working position with correction carried out in the final detailing of the occlusion.

Commercial plastic devices are available which can assist in bite registration (Fig. 5.8). These must be buried in the wax wafer and have a notch to engage the upper incisors and several

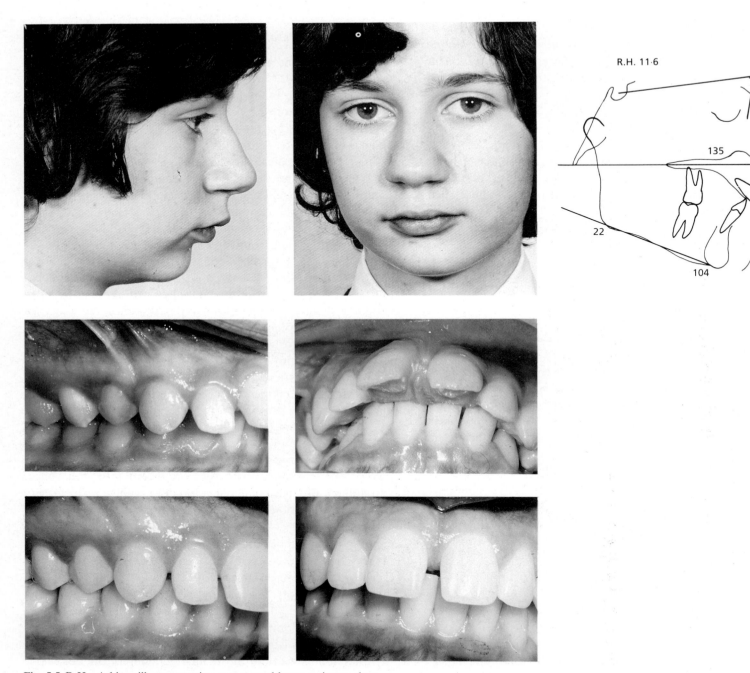

Fig. 5.5 R.H.: A bimaxillary protrusion case treated by an activator alone.

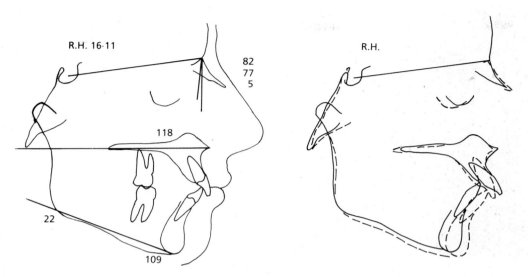

Fig. 5.5 (*cont'd*)

notches for the lowers. These devices do not allow variation in incisor separation and may not suit all cases.

At this stage it is important to give clear instructions to the laboratory for the design of the chosen appliance.

Fitting appliances

The appliance should be shown to the patient on the models so that its mode of action can be explained. The appliance is then fitted and a careful check is made to ensure that there are no sources of local pressure or discomfort. With a hand mirror the patient is shown the appliance in the mouth and removal and replacement of the appliance is demonstrated. The patient can practise fitting the appliance using a wall-mounted mirror.

INSTRUCTIONS FOR WEAR

Initially the patient is expected to wear the appliance for approximately 6 hours each day, for a training period of 2 weeks.

With the minimal bulk appliances which are expected to be worn virtually full-time, the patient is asked to read aloud with the appliance in the mouth for a period each day, so that at the end of the training period they should be able to speak reasonably well with the appliance fitted.

At the end of the 2-week period the patient should be seen again and adjustments should be made if any discomfort has arisen. The patient is then encouraged to wear the appliance for the appropriate amount of time each day, and during sleep. The importance of wearing the appliance for the maximum number of hours each day should be stressed, with the proviso that the appliance should be left out for any active games, or sports.

It is psychologically important to avoid the use of the term 'night-time brace' or 'part-time brace'. To encourage patient motivation and to involve them in the treatment, charts can be issued to the patients on which they can record the hours of the day that the appliance is worn and can calculate a daily average of wear (Fig. 5.9). Verbal instructions given to the patient and parent should be reinforced by the provision of printed instructions, thus:

INSTRUCTIONS FOR PATIENTS

1 The appliance that you have been given works by stretching the muscles of the jaws. For the first 2 weeks it should be worn

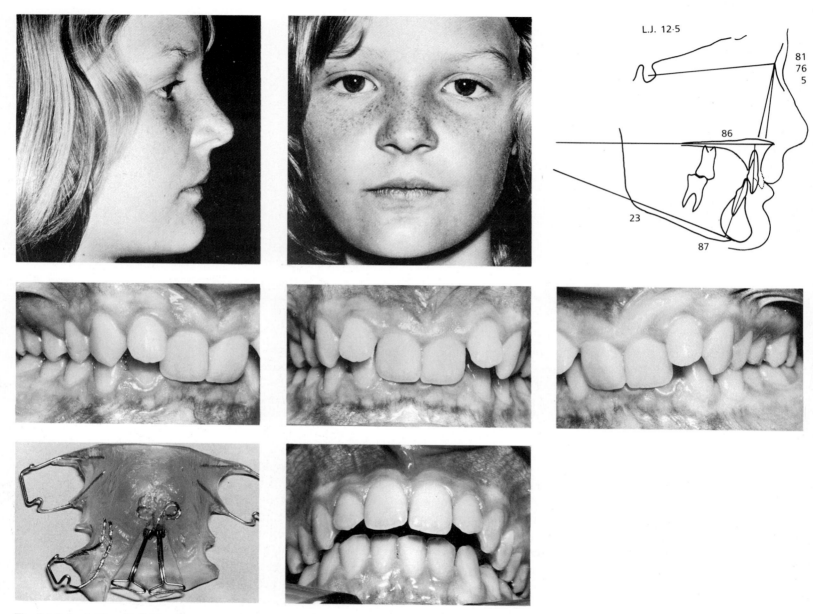

Fig. 5.6 L.J.: A Class II division 2 case treated by proclination of the upper incisors with a removable appliance, followed by Class II correction with a functional appliance. This case was stable 5 years out of retention and after the third molars were removed.

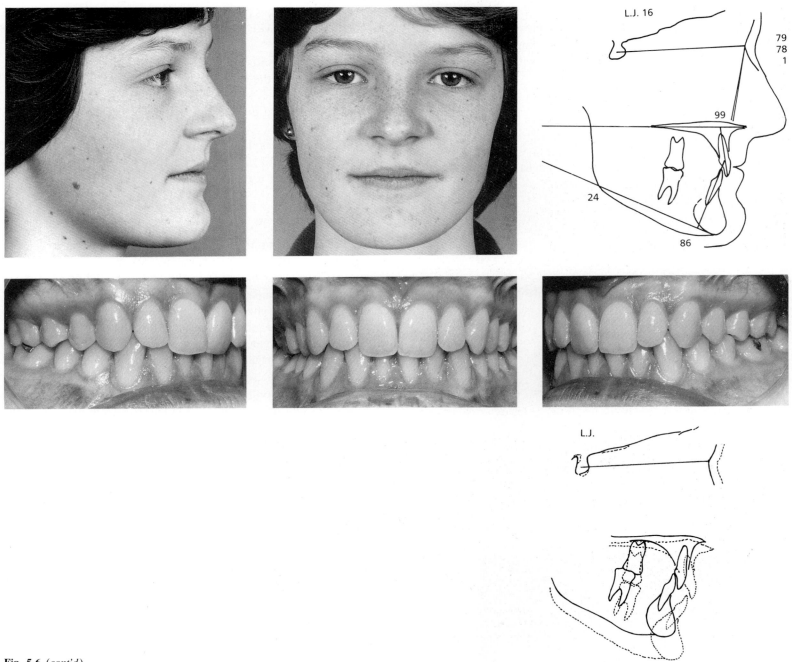

Fig. 5.6 (*cont'd*)

for a total of 6 hours a day. You will probably manage this between coming home from school and before going to bed.

2 During this training period practice reading aloud for 10 minutes each day. This will help you to talk with the appliance in your mouth.

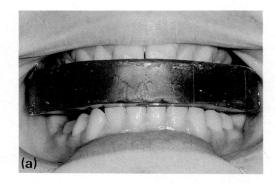

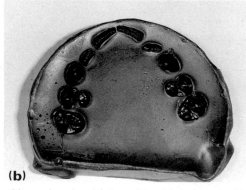

Fig. 5.7 A wax bite registration (a) in position in the mouth, (b) showing indentations of the maxillary teeth.

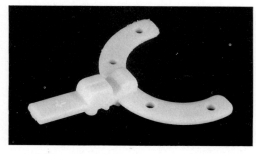

Fig. 5.8 A commercially produced bite fork.

3 After two weeks you will have an appointment with your orthodontist who will check that the brace is not rubbing or causing discomfort.

4 Provided all is satisfactory, once the training period is over, wear the brace all the time including going to school and whilst asleep.

5 When eating and during games and sport leave the appliance in a box.

6 If the appliance is damaged, broken or uncomfortable contact your orthodontist for an early appointment and if possible try to continue wearing it for some time each day.

Assessment of progress

When the patient enters the surgery it is important to ask whether they have experienced any problems with the wear of the appliance. The patient is seated in the chair and asked to demonstrate that he is familiar with removing and fitting the appliance. Where appropriate check to see that the patient can speak with the appliance in the mouth. The appliance should then be examined for signs of wear. These may be facets caused by occlusal contact with the acrylic or calculus on various parts of the appliance. The patient should then be asked to produce the time charts so that the hours of wear can be discussed with them. It is then wise to measure the patient's height so that any change from the last visit can be recorded on the height chart.

Occlusal assessment

The overjet should be measured, taking care to ensure that the patient has the mandible in the maximum retruded position. Where progress is good it is often found that the patients find it extremely difficult to achieve maximum retrusion without discomfort. Another sign of successful wear is often the development of a slight lateral openbite. The overbite should be assessed and the molar relationship should be compared with the situation on the original study models. Depending upon the appliances used, other specific dental measurements may be made using dividers and ruler. Accurate records of all the findings should be made in the patient's clinical notes with special reference to changes that have taken place.

If the patient's progress is satisfactory a new appointment can be made for further checking of the appliance after 6 to 8 weeks,

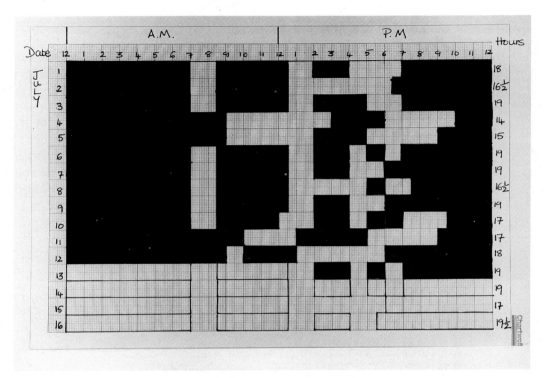

Fig. 5.9 A time chart illustrating daily hours of wear.

depending upon the appliance being used. This process of careful assessment must be made at each subsequent appointment.

Unsatisfactory progress

Within two to three visits significant clinical change should be seen; if this is not so, then it is wise to check carefully the patient's time chart and also to record a height measurement. If he or she has grown, the height chart should be shown to the patient, with an explanation that an increase in height should be accompanied by a reduction in overjet, provided the appliance has been worn for a sufficient period of time each day. The importance of wearing the appliance as much as possible should be stressed to the patient. Where progress is slow it is important to tell the parent so that they can assist in encouraging the patient to persevere with the appliance.

Because there is always an element of doubt about co-operation when using functional appliances, it is wise to make a firm rule to review the treatment within 6 months of commencement. If progress is unsatisfactory it is sensible to reassess the treatment plan at this stage.

Reactivation

Reactivation is required in many cases before treatment is completed. A sure sign that reactivation is indicated is a significant reduction of the overjet. With many appliances it is often possible to check whether reactivation is necessary by asking the patient to disengage the lower teeth from the appliance, and seeing if the mandible can be postured significantly further forwards. Even if there has not been a particularly large reduction of overjet, patients who are co-operating with their appliances can usually posture their mandibles significantly further forwards than they could before treatment started and so re-activation is beneficial.

Completion of functional appliance treatment

Following completion of functional appliance treatment there are three options:
1 Retain with the existing appliance which may need to be modified.
2 Retain with an alternative appliance.
3 Complete treatment with another appliance system.

Retention with functional appliance

This may easily be achieved by reducing the time of wear of the appliance to nights only to maintain the class II effect which should be continued until the growth spurt is completed. This should be confirmed by standing height records. Some appliances may require modification to allow a satisfactory intercuspation to develop.

Retention with an alternative appliance

At the end of treatment, as with any orthodontic case a removable retainer such as a Hawley, or Begg, retainer may be used. In a Class II case there is a possibility that despite this the overjet may tend to relapse and therefore it may be wise to incorporate headgear to the appliance on a nights only basis.

Change to other appliance systems

Treatment may frequently need to be completed by a combination of fixed appliances and headgear. In a Class II case when the functional appliance is discarded in order to change over to a fixed appliance it is wise to maintain a distal force to the upper arch, usually by means of headgear. Without this there is a tendency for the upper arch position to relapse once the functional element of treatment is removed. The lower arch must be bracketed to maintain overbite control. The appointment for the placement of separators must be made while the functional appliance is still being worn.

References

Loh, N.K. & Kerr, W.J.S. (1985) The FR 3. Effects and Indications. *British Journal of Orthodontics*, **12**, 153.

Morndal, O. (1984) The effects on incisor teeth of activator treatment. *British Journal of Orthodontics*, **11**, 214.

Further reading

Cohen, A. (1981) Class II division 1 malocclusion treated by Andresen appliance. *British Journal of Orthodontics*, **8**, 159.

Graber, T.M. & Neuman, B. (1977) Removable appliance orthodontics. W.B. Saunders, Philadelphia.

Proffit, W.R. (1985) Determinants of success with functional appliance treatment. In: Graber, T.M. (ed.), *Physiologic Principles of Functional Appliances*, Ch. 10. Mosby, St Louis.

Chapter 6   The Appliances

The Andresen appliance

Andresen is credited with the introduction of the concept of functional orthodontic treatment, although Robin, in France, described a similar method somewhat earlier. By the second decade of this century Andresen had published numerous articles in the European literature describing his techniques and, in 1939, published his book with Haupl, *Funktions-Kieferorthopadie*. The appliance described by Andresen is probably still the best known of all functional appliances and has been described in many standard orthodontic text books.

The principal action of the Andresen appliance is dento-alveolar tooth movement particularly of the upper incisors, often with favourable change in the molar occlusion from Class II to Class I. Claims for significant change in skeletal pattern have been difficult to substantiate. Most investigators confirm that tooth movement is achieved principally by dento-alveolar change with at best only a most modest improvement in the underlying skeletal structures.

Design of the appliance

The appliance is constructed from acrylic with the base plate covering the palate and the lingual aspect of the lower ridge with shallow lingual flanges. The appliance has a labial bow anterior to the upper incisors which is usually fairly inflexible although there are U-loops for adjustment (Fig. 6.1). In its original form the appliance contacts the lower anterior teeth only on the lingual side and does not cover the incisal edges or any part of the labial surface. The acrylic is relieved on the palatal aspect of the upper anterior teeth. The chief distinguishing feature of the appliance is the buccal faceting which is so designed as to direct the movement of the teeth in the buccal segments (Fig. 6.2). On the upper surface, these facets are cut so as to allow the occlusal, distal and buccal movement of these teeth. This is achieved by keeping the acrylic in contact only with the mesio-palatal surface of the premolars and molars. On the lower, these facets only permit upward and forward movement with the acrylic contacting the disto-lingual aspect of the teeth (Fig. 6.3). The facets are not produced in the laboratory, but are created at the chairside by the clinician. The appliance is delivered from the laboratory to the clinic with a clear imprint of the palatal and occlusal surfaces of the buccal teeth reflected in the acrylic. It is a time-consuming chairside procedure to trim the appliance and create the correct facets. Practitioners experienced in the use of this appliance claim that the correct manipulation of the buccal part of these appliances plays an important role in the correction of the buccal occlusion.

Over many years of experience in using this appliance a number of clinicians have described modifications to its original design. One of the main modifications was developed by Rix (1966), who

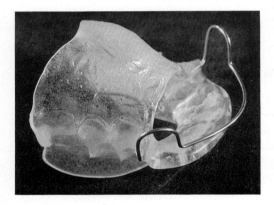

Fig. 6.1 An Andresen appliance.

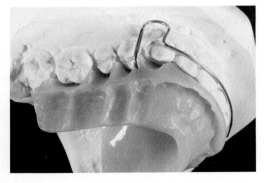

Fig. 6.2 Buccal facets are cut to encourage disto-buccal movement of upper buccal teeth and to allow mesial movement of lower buccal teeth.

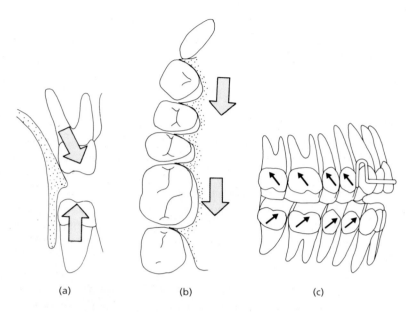

Fig. 6.3 The appliance is trimmed to encourage: (a) buccal movement of the upper teeth; (b) distal movement of the upper teeth; (c) mesial movement of the lower teeth and an intrusive component of force on the upper teeth.

introduced an airhole into the appliance to enable those with frequent upper respiratory tract infections to be able to tolerate the appliance. Other principal modifications have been:
1 The addition of screws in the midline to create upper arch expansion.
2 Springs for individual tooth movement.
3 Modification to the labial bow.

Clinical considerations

The Andresen appliance was originally intended to treat Class II division 1 malocclusions. In addition to being suitable for treating those patients who had difficulty in attending regular appointments because of the distances involved, Andresen considered that the appliance achieved a more physiological approach to orthodontic therapy than that resulting from the fixed appliances used at that time (Schmuth 1983). However, in common with all removable appliances, the Andresen is not able to carry out independent alignment of more than one or two teeth at a time or simultaneously to change the positions of individual teeth. The Andresen is used mainly in malocclusions which demonstrate

only a moderate severity in their Class II element with no crowding or irregularity in either arch. There is no doubt that in clinical practice the Andresen appliance can be very effective in the treatment of such malocclusions and many papers have been published demonstrating this.

One of the features of the appliance which has been the focus of considerable attention is its tendency to procline the lower incisor teeth. Because the lingual flanges are small, most of the Class II force generated by the appliance is applied through the lower dentition. There is an inevitable tendency for forward movement of the teeth in this arch and the teeth most likely to move are the incisors. It is for this reason that a number of clinicians have suggested that only those cases demonstrating spacing of the lower arch at the start of treatment are suitable for Andresen appliance treatment. This spacing is to allow for the relapse of the lower anterior teeth back to their pre-treatment angulation after appliances are withdrawn without resultant crowding. However, a number of authors have demonstrated that proclination of the lower labial segment is not a constant feature of Andresen appliance therapy.

Malocclusions other than Class II division 1 have been successfully treated by the Andresen appliance. Mild Class II division 2 malocclusions are occasionally treated by proclining the upper central incisors to convert the malocclusion into a type of Class II division 1 which is then treated with an Andresen appliance.

Some clinicians have occasionally advocated the use of the Andresen appliance in the treatment of Class III malocclusions. Here the appliance must be modified to include an active component because it is not possible to posture the mandible significantly backwards. This is accomplished by constructing the appliance in separate mandibular and maxillary halves and incorporating a screw between them. This can be turned to advance the upper part relative to the lower part to aid in the correction of the Class III relationship. However, even the most enthusiastic advocates of functional appliance therapy would probably agree that there are more efficient ways of dealing with the limited number of Class III malocclusions which respond to functional appliance treatment.

VERTICAL CONSIDERATIONS

In its original form the Andresen appliance is not particularly suited to malocclusions which demonstrate a significant increase in incisor overbite. This is because the lack of acrylic cover over the lower incisal edges does not permit a bite plane effect. Conversely, when an anterior openbite is present, especially when associated with a sucking habit, an Andresen appliance can be very useful. Provision of such an appliance is often helpful to patients who have a mild Class II division 1 malocclusion and are endeavouring to abandon a habit.

RADIAL CONSIDERATIONS

Where there is a pre-existing buccal crossbite associated with a lateral displacement it is usually advisable to correct this with a removable appliance before commencing Andresen treatment. If this is likely to delay the functional stage of treatment beyond the age of maximum growth then it is advisable to commence with the Andresen straightaway, in which case it is important to ensure that the mandible is not in its laterally displaced position when the bite is taken. During treatment the addition of cold-cure acrylic to the palatal contacts with the upper posterior teeth may help to encourage the necessary increase in upper arch width.

It has often been suggested that it is necessary to expand maxillary arches when correcting Class II malocclusions with a functional appliance so that the intermolar width will increase during treatment. This is intended to preserve a correct buccolingual relationship of upper and lower molars and avoid the creation of unwanted crossbites during sagittal correction. For this reason a number of clinicians have advocated the incorporation of a coffin spring or screw in the midline. As the appliance is divided in the sagittal plane into left and right halves, the problem with this arrangement is that the appliance also acts on the lower arch and may cause unnecessary lower arch expansion.

COMBINATION TREATMENT

As a consequence of the close fit of the facets to the posterior teeth it is not convenient to use such an appliance in association with fixed appliances, although these may be used after the Andresen treatment is complete. Headgear may be readily applied to the appliance either by a face bow fitting into tubes in the appliance, or by J-hooks engaging hooks on the labial bow embedded into the acrylic.

Due to the need to select cases which do not show significant crowding or irregularity, Andresen appliance therapy is not used in conjunction with extractions, with the exception of the enforced loss of first permanent molars prior to the commencement of treatment.

Management of the appliance

The appliance must be constructed from adequate upper and lower impressions and an accurate working occlusal registration. Generally the mandible is postured 2–3 mm forwards and downwards from the resting position, taking care to keep the centre lines coincident. The technician then constructs the appliance in heat-cured acrylic to the working bite registration using unadjusted working models from the original impressions. The appliance is then delivered to the clinician for trimming and fitting. Some clinicians choose to leave the appliance untrimmed at the first visit believing that in this state it will be more retentive and thereby enable the patient to become more rapidly used to its presence. The chief modification to the method of trimming is to be seen in the lower arch. Here, although classically the guiding facets are fashioned to encourage forward and upward movement in the lower posterior teeth, it is felt by some that this is an undesirable aspect of Andresen appliance therapy. Such people maintain that all interdental facets in the lower arch should be removed so that the teeth are free to erupt and move mesially but are not actively encouraged to do so (Fig. 6.4). This modification can be seen as a stage in the evolution of the activator of Harvold.

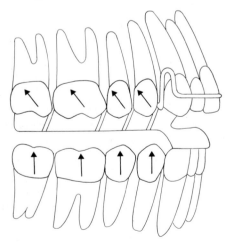

Fig. 6.4 The lower acrylic trimmed away to allow for the eruption of the lower teeth. In the upper arch acrylic contact restrains vertical development.

The Andresen appliance is intended to be a loose-fitting appliance and most patients tolerate it fairly readily, although it is not possible to speak or eat with the appliance in place and most workers therefore regard the appliance as being essentially a part-time appliance. Because of its bulk and relatively loose-fitting design, the appliance is at first prone to be rejected when the patient is asleep. After the usual training period these difficulties are usually overcome.

The appliance can be used in the mixed or early permanent dentition. Considerable modification may be required as the deciduous teeth are shed and replaced by the permanent successors. Adjustments can be made to the buccal facets by careful trimming or the addition of very small quantities of cold-cure acrylic. Because of the need for the appliance to be in close contact with teeth in the buccal segments, when more than a small number of deciduous teeth have been shed the construction of a new appliance is usually necessary. Otherwise, fundamental reactivation of the appliance cannot be achieved without the provision of a new one. It is common in Andresen therapy for two or more appliances to be required to complete the necessary tooth movements.

RETENTION

There are no specific requirements for retention following Andresen appliance therapy and there is no need to construct formal retainers. It is advisable, however, to be cautious in the immediate post-treatment period. Most operators prefer to remove the facets in the final stages of treatment to ensure the establishment of a satisfactory buccal intercuspation. When satisfactory tooth movement has been achieved it is wise to withdraw the appliance slowly over some months by asking the patient to reduce the wear by degrees, finishing by wearing it only one or two nights per week. At this point the appliance can be finally abandoned and suitable records taken to monitor future changes.

References

Andresen, V. & Haupl, K. (1939) *Funktions-Kieferorthopadie*, Meusser, Leipzig.
Schmuth, G.P.F. (1983) Milestones in the development and practical application of functional appliances. *American Journal of Orthodontics*, **84**, 48.

Further reading

Calvert, F.J. (1982) An assessment of Andresen therapy on Class II division 1 malocclusions. *British Journal of Orthodontics*, **9**, 149.
Parkhouse, R.C. (1968) Cephalometric appraisal of Angle's Class II division 1 malocclusion treated by the Andresen appliance. *Transactions of the British Society for the Study of Orthodontics*, **55**, 61.
Reichborn-Kjyennerud, A.M. (1973) Andresen's conception of functional jaw orthopaedics. *Transactions of European Orthodontic Society* 215.
Rix, R.E. (1966) Further thoughts on monobloc therapy. *Transactions of the British Society for the Study of Orthodontics*, **53**, 1.
Robertson, N.R.E. (1963) The Andresen appliance in the treatment of Angle class II division 1 malocclusions. *British Dental Journal*, **114**, 262–264.
Robin, P. (1902) Demonstration pratique sur la construction et la mise en bouche d'un nouvel appareil de redressment. *Revue de stomatologie*, **IX**, 36.
Trayfoot, J. & Richardson, A. (1968) Angle Class II division 1 malocclusions treated by the Andresen method. *British Dental Journal*, **124**, 516.

The activator

The activator is probably the most widely used derivative of Andresen's original appliance. Most of the credit for the development of the activator must go to Harvold who, following his experience in Norway with the Andresen appliance, moved to North America. There he suggested a number of modifications to the Andresen in order to overcome some of the shortcomings of the original appliance and to increase its clinical scope. From these modifications the modern activator has developed and it is this appliance that the authors find to be the most useful of all functional appliances in the management of Class II cases (Fig. 6.5).

As well as introducing these modifications, Harvold proposed in his text book 'The Activator in Interceptive Orthodontics' (1974) that the role of the appliance should be widened. Rather than selecting a small group of cases which might respond satisfactorily to functional appliance therapy, Harvold suggested that the activator should be used across a broad spectrum of Class II cases as an interceptive device. Problems which would be regarded as contra-indications to the use of the Andresen appliance, such as severe Class 2 skeletal pattern, crowding, absence of teeth, or local tooth malpositioning, merely dictated the need for a second phase of treatment. Usually, this involves fixed appliance techniques (see below). The activator's role in this regimen is to correct the incisor overjet and overbite and the molar relationship during a period of active facial growth.

Clinical experience with this appliance has led us to believe

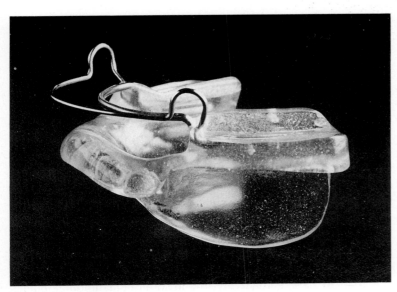

Fig. 6.5 The activator.

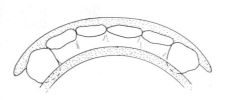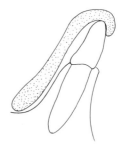

Fig. 6.6 Design of the lower incisor capping.

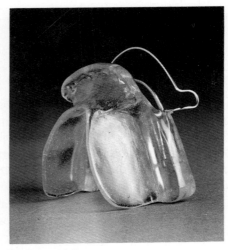

Fig. 6.7 The extended lingual flanges.

that it is more effective in influencing the growth and development of the underlying skeletal pattern than an Andresen appliance. While this may be demonstrated in a number of successfully treated cases, it has to be admitted that longitudinal studies of consecutively treated cases still leave open the question as to whether or not the activator significantly influences the growth of the facial bones, and whether it is any more effective than any other variety of functional appliance.

Design of the appliance

The main modifications from an Andresen appliance for a Class II activator are as follows:

1 Extension of the lower anterior acrylic over the incisal edges and on to the labial surfaces of the lower incisors in an attempt to limit the tendency of the appliance to procline the lower anterior teeth (Fig. 6.6).

2 Maximum extension of the lower lingual flanges in order to redistribute as much of the Class II force as possible on to the mucoperiostium of the mandible (Fig. 6.7).

3 The design of the appliance in the buccal segments involves a totally different concept to that of the Andresen. Occlusal shelves which are flat contact the cusp tips of the upper buccal segment

teeth. This is in contrast with the interdental facets of the Andresen which are designed to guide the eruption of the upper teeth distally and buccally at the same time as the lower teeth are guided mesially. The occlusal shelf does not have any contact at all with the lower posterior teeth, the aim of the appliance being to adjust the occlusal plane by a restriction of downward and forward eruption of the maxillary teeth, and to allow upward and forward development of the lower posterior teeth, thus changing a Class II to a Class I molar relationship (Fig. 6.8).

4 By comparison with other functional appliances there is a considerable increase in the vertical dimension of the appliance which is achieved by taking a working occlusal registration extending well beyond the freeway space. This bite registration should give a separation of the anterior teeth of the order of 1 cm as opposed to the 2−3 mm associated with an Andresen appliance.

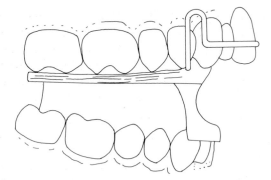

Fig. 6.8 The occlusal shelves contact the upper molar cusp tips—they must be kept clear of the lower posterior teeth.

Clinical considerations

The activator, like the Andresen appliance, is almost exclusively used in the treatment of Class II division 1 malocclusions for which it is ideally suited. It is particularly effective at reducing increased incisor overbites because of the influence of the occlusal shelf on the upper molars and the incisal capping which prevents vertical development of the lower incisors, whilst the occlusal shelves allow for development of the lower buccal teeth. The large vertical dimension of the appliance enhances this effect. This gives rise to a relative increase in facial height and overbite reduction. It can therefore treat a large range of Class II division 1 malocclusions with average to low maxillary mandibular planes angle and associated deep bites. A small but significant proportion of malocclusions of this type which show good arch alignment at the commencement of treatment, whether in the mixed or permanent dentition, can be treated solely with an activator without requiring a finishing phase of fixed appliance therapy. Nevertheless, by the standards of present day orthodontic treatment, many cases would require such finishing in order to effect detailed tooth positioning and enhance the stability of the result.

Class II division 2 cases can be treated using the activator provided that an initial phase using a removable or fixed appliance has achieved satisfactory upper incisor alignment by converting the incisor relationship from Class II division 2 to Class II division 1. It is useful if the overbite can be reduced during this phase of treatment and for this reason an upper removable appliance with an anterior bite plane is particularly appropriate. The activator is then constructed as for the treatment of a Class II division 1 malocclusion except that acrylic is not relieved behind the palatal surface of the upper incisors but is kept in contact with them in order to maintain the proclination achieved by the first phase of treatment.

Many attempts have been made to influence Class III malocclusions using the activator. Since one of the chief features of the activator is to control the upper and lower buccal segments, the construction of the occlusal flanges is the opposite to that recommended for Class II malocclusions. In Class III cases it is the upper buccal teeth which are free from occlusal contact with the acrylic and allowed free downwards and forwards movement due to natural eruptive forces whilst the lower posterior teeth are prevented from moving by contact of the cusps with the occlusal shelf. Such buccal tooth manipulation is only appropriate in members of that group of Class III cases which demonstrate significant incisor overbite at the commencement of treatment and tend to have a relatively low maxillary–mandibular planes angle. Class III cases which exhibit a reduced incisor overbite are not appropriate for activator therapy and are best treated entirely with conventional dento-alveolar tooth movements or orthognatic surgery. It would seem therefore that the number of Class III cases appropriate for treatment with this appliance is relatively small.

VERTICAL CONTROL

The activator is particularly effective in the reduction of overbites, and cases exhibiting low maxillary–mandibular planes angle with excessive overbite are well suited to the appliance. The appliance is not, however, efficient at controlling the vertical position of the upper labial segments.

Management of high-angle cases and openbites, as with most other appliance systems, is more difficult. The occlusal shelves are modified in order to reduce vertical development of the posterior teeth and thus avoid excessive face height increase and backward rotation of the mandible. This is achieved by making the occlusal shelf contact the cusp tips of the lower posterior teeth in addition to the normal contact with the upper posterior teeth. The lower incisors are not capped and the acrylic lingual to them is replaced by a stainless steel bar. This is to ensure that the teeth are free to develop vertically. Such combination of inhibition of the molar development and free vertical development of both the upper and the lower incisors encourages closure of an anterior openbite (Fig. 6.9).

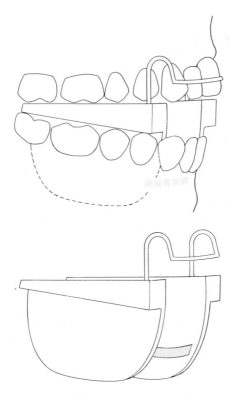

Fig. 6.9 An appliance for a high-angle case with a stainless steel lingual bar.

RADIAL CONSIDERATIONS

Where there is a unilateral or bilateral buccal crossbite the authors' preference is to treat this first with a suitable expansion appliance prior to constructing and fitting the activator. In cases which do not exhibit crossbites it is not necessary to carry out any preliminary expansion either with a separate appliance beforehand or with a modified functional appliance. Increase in molar width occurs to maintain a correct bucco-lingual relationship of the upper and lower molars as the Class II antero-posterior relationship is improved. The reason for this is unknown, but the occlusal shelves allow free movement of the molars which may result from normal growth and cuspal forces during function. Operators who use Adams clasps to aid retention of the appliance may find that a crossbite develops as the intermolar width is held by the appliance. If clasps are used they should be removed from the appliance once the patient is accustomed to wearing it.

Crowding of the dentition is also rather easier to manage than with the Andresen appliance as premolar extractions can be carried out before or during appliance therapy. In some cases spontaneous tooth movement within each arch (Fig. 6.10) can achieve some or all of the necessary space closure during and after the active phase of functional appliance treatment. Nevertheless, it is inevitable that a proportion of extraction cases will require completion with fixed appliances.

COMBINATION TREATMENT

One of the advantages of the activator is its ability to be used in conjunction with other appliance systems. Since the acrylic of the appliance is not in intimate contact with the teeth it is possible to place bands and brackets to carry out other tooth movements while the activator is being worn. During the initial phase of treatment it is often appropriate to place bands on upper first molars and in some cases to add headgear. Assistance with overbite control can be achieved by fitting a lower fixed appliance with the appropriate arch wires to intrude the incisors and or assist in the vertical development of the lower buccal teeth. When the time comes to complete the functional aspect of treatment a smooth transition can be made from this stage to the full bracketed appliance to achieve any necessary finishing tooth movements.

Management of the appliance

Because the activator has deeply extended lingual flanges it is essential to have good working impressions. Many mistakes have been made by failing to appreciate this and it may be helpful on occasion to use a special tray for the lower arch in order to get an accurate representation of the lingual mucoperiostium. The working occlusal registration is taken by displacement of the mandible considerably further open than the classical Andresen

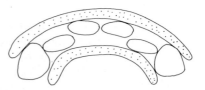

Fig. 6.10 The lower incisor capping is designed to allow distal movement of canines and relief of lower crowding.

teaching. Specially constructed wax bite blocks approximately 10 mm thick assist this registration.

At the time of fitting it is important to explain to the patient and the parent the nature of the appliance as its large size can be somewhat surprising. When fitting the appliance for the first time it is important to do so by engaging the lower arch first and then asking the patient to posture the mandible sufficiently forwards to enable the labial wire to be positioned against the buccal surface of the upper anterior teeth. If an attempt is made to insert the appliance in the reverse fashion by first engaging the upper teeth it will usually be impossible to seat the mandibular dentition correctly because the lingual flanges are unable to gain their correct position in the lingual undercut. Despite occasional initial difficulties, a high proportion of patients tolerate the appliance very well and if it is properly constructed it is much better retained in the mouth than the more loose-fitting Andresen appliance. In cases where subconscious night-time rejection occurs it is helpful to increase the retentive possibilities by adding headgear to the appliance or appropriate retentive clasps. The appliance is initially difficult to wear full-time, and patients find a degree of interference with speech, but most patients can soon speak adequately with the appliance in the mouth and should therefore be encourage to wear the appliance at school. Like all other functional appliances it should be worn as much as possible with an aim to achieve between 14 and 20 hours a day. Experienced practitioners can often motivate their good patients to wear the activator full-time, which leads to an improved clinical response. At the first visit following the fitting of the appliance, some easing of the lingual flange may be necessary. If possible this should be achieved by reducing the thickness of the flange rather than by reducing its length. The use of easing wax helps to avoid this mistake.

OCCLUSAL MANAGEMENT

The standard measurements of overjet and overbite should be recorded at each visit, as well as noting change in the molar relationship. With good wear 1 to 2 mm of overjet reduction should be seen between visits. When checking the overjet, ensure that the patient is not posturing forwards. It will often be discovered that the patient finds it extremely uncomfortable to get into maximum retrusion. This is an encouraging sign and is usually associated with rapid improvement in the occlusion. A lateral

openbite also develops where sagittal correction is progressing rapidly. Because the appliance is fairly rigid the appointments can be made at 6—8-week intervals, unless encouragement and reinforcement is required.

Activator therapy can be instituted at any time in the development of the dentition but will need to be continued until at least peak growth has passed. It is generally advantageous to commence during the mixed dentition stage. Since there are no detailed facets to contact the buccal teeth, the deciduous teeth are shed and replaced by permanent successors without having to remake the appliance.

In order to take advantage of a period of active growth it will be necessary to reactivate the appliance during treatment. This is very much simpler than when using the Andresen appliance and can best be achieved by separating the maxillary and mandibular halves horizontally and reuniting them with the mandible postured further forward as the clinical requirements dictate (Fig. 6.11). The activator can be sectioned horizontally at the level of the occlusal shelf with a bur, or better still a fret saw. The two halves can be reunited in a number of ways. A new bite registration can be taken directly in the mouth or, with experience, the halves can be reunited directly with cold-cure acrylic in the mouth. Alternatively an experienced technician can carry out all the necessary advancement 'on the bench' providing he has been given an indication of the advancement required. Refitting the reactivated appliance usually presents no difficulty.

RETENTION

Where the activator has been used alone then gradual reduction in the hours of wear is the first step towards dispensing with the appliance completely. If the occlusal change has been particularly rapid it is wise to continue retention on a nights only basis until it is certain that the growth spurt is completed. It is also usual to remove the occlusal shelves at this stage so that the posterior teeth can achieve full intercuspation (Fig. 6.12). This is particularly important if some of the permanent teeth have yet to erupt. When treatment is completed with fixed appliances then the usual guidelines for post-treatment retention can be adhered to. However some Class II or headgear force should again be maintained until the growth spurt has been passed.

If there is concern that the lower labial segment has been proclined excessively then it is possible to ease the lingual acrylic

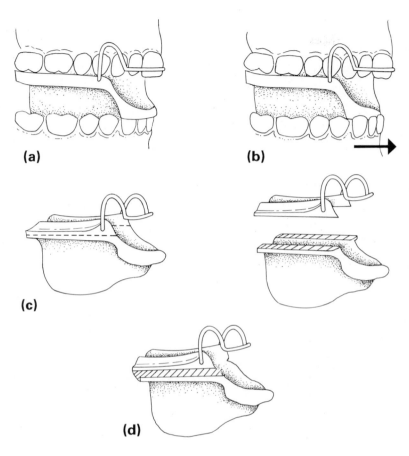

Fig. 6.11 Reactivation of an activator. (a) The appliance in position; (b) the patient can posture anterior to the capping; (c) the appliance is then cut into two halves; (d) the halves are reunited in the new forward position.

away from the lower incisor contact, or indeed to remove this section completely.

Reference

Harvold, E.P. (1974) *The Activator in Interceptive Orthodontics*. Mosby, St Louis.

Further reading

Harvold, E.P. & Vargervik, K. (1971) Morphogenetic response to activator treatment. *American Journal of Orthodontics*, **60**, 478.
Isaacson, K.G., Reed, R.T. & Stephens, C.D. (1983) Simplified construction and use of the Activator. *Journal of Clinical Orthodontics*, **17**, 845.

Reed, R.T. & Hathorn, I.S (1978). The Activator. *British Journal of Orthodontics*, **5**, 75.
Stephens, C.D., Isaacson, K.G. & Reed, R.T. (1984) The modified Activator. *Journal of Clinical Orthodontics*, **18**, 650.
Vargervik, K. & Harvold, E.P. (1985) Response to activator treatment in Class II malocclusions. *American Journal of Orthodontics*, **88**, 242.
Woodside, D.G., (1977) In: Graber, T.M. & Neumann, B. (eds) *The Activator in Removable Orthodontic Appliances*. W.B. Saunders, Philadelphia.

The bionator

The appliance was developed in the 1950s by Balters, who lay considerable stress on the importance of the tongue in the development of openbites and Class II and Class III malocclusions.

It is a light appliance with minimum bulk and as it is relatively easy to speak with the appliance in the mouth it can therefore be worn virtually full-time. The original aim of the appliance was to bring the tongue into its correct position, and thus encourage normal development of the arches rather than to stretch and activate the facial muscles and muscles of mastication as a means of producing dentofacial change.

Design of the appliance

The appliance consists of a lingual horseshoe of acrylic, with a palatal spring which is shaped like a reversed coffin spring which passes distally over the palate, but does not contact the palatal mucosa: there are facets in the acrylic which accept the posterior teeth in the maxillary and mandibular arches and hold these in a postured relationship. The facets extend to cover approximately half the bucco-lingual width of the posterior teeth and, although these contact the posterior teeth, the relatively loose fit of the appliance makes control of tooth position by eruptive guidance quite difficult. The labial bow is placed just clear of the incisors and is extended distally where it is designed to keep the cheeks away from the buccal aspect of the teeth (Fig. 6.13). The appliance is made with the mandible positioned forwards until there is virtually an edge-to-edge incisor relationship (see below). This is to prevent the tongue from posturing forwards and maintaining an increased overjet.

Clinical considerations

The appliance is ideally suited for the management of mild Class II division 1 occlusions, especially those that do not exhibit crowd-

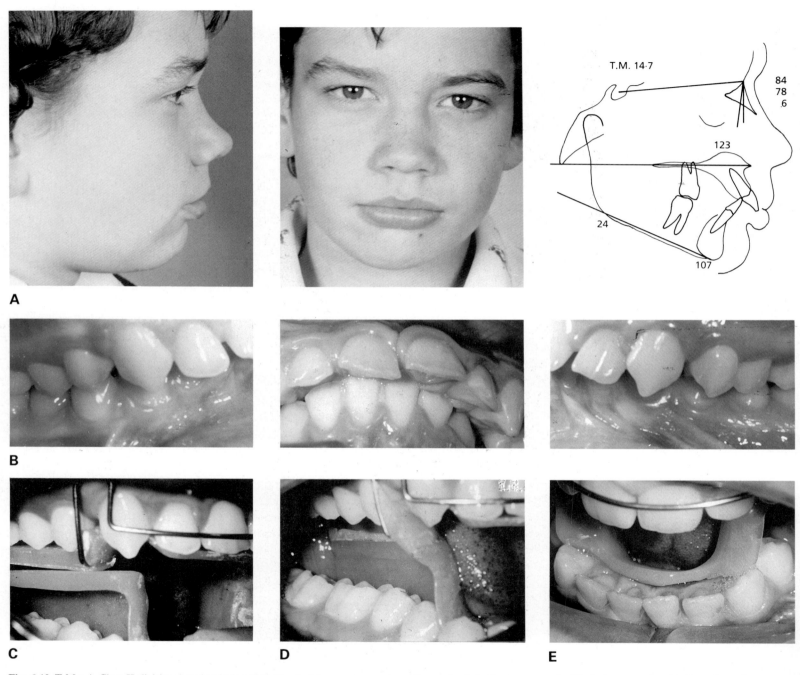

Fig. 6.12 T.M.: A Class II division 1 malocclusion. (A) The facial appearance at the start of treatment; (B) the initial occlusion with a traumatic overbite and an overjet of 11 mm; (C) during treatment the activator was split and is shown in the advanced position prior to uniting the two halves together; (D) during retention the occlusal shelf was removed; (E) during retention the lingual acrylic was removed from behind the lower incisors; (F) the facial appearance 2 years out of retention. The patient declined fixed appliances for alignment and closure of the diastema.

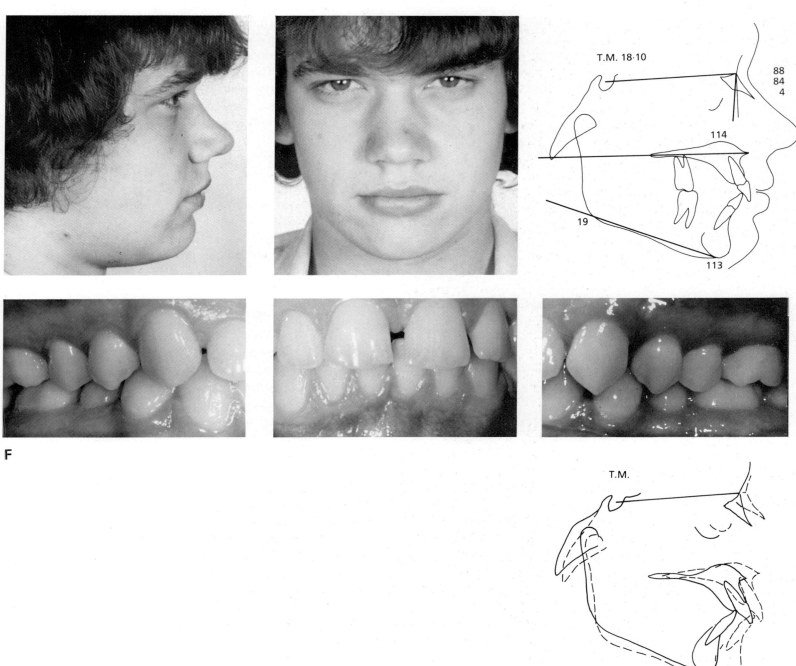

F

Fig. 6.12 (*cont'd*)

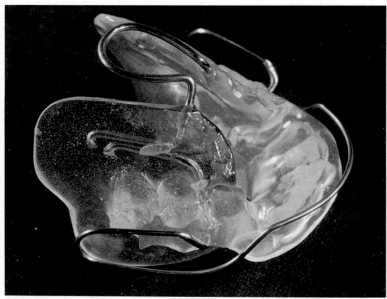

Fig. 6.13 A bionator.

ing. Most of the change achieved with the bionator is dento-alveolar. For this reason and also because it is constructed with the incisors in an edge-to-edge position it is not as suitable for more marked Class 2 skeletal patterns as is the activator. The appliance has various modifications, with specific designs for open-bite and Class III occlusions. The correction of Class II division 2 occlusions is not easily achieved because of the problem of overbite and the difficulty in maintaining the proclination of the upper incisors. Lower incisor proclination seems to occur fairly readily with the appliance, therefore only cases without crowding are suitable for treatment. Modifications described by Ellisdon & Hunt (1985) include versions with incisor capping and trimming of the acrylic lingual to the lower incisors. They also recommend complete removal of any occlusal contact in the buccal region with only minimal guidance to the premolar and molar teeth.

VERTICAL CONSIDERATIONS

Even though the appliance can be made with acrylic covering of the incisal edges, correction of excessive overbite is difficult and overbite correction is achieved by relative change in eruption rates of the posterior teeth once the overjet reduction has been

achieved. A specific appliance design is used for anterior openbite cases. In this the incisors are brought as close to edge-to-edge as possible and the resultant space is obliterated by an extension of the lingual acrylic. The aim of this is to prevent continued tongue thrusting. As the treatment progresses, the acrylic has to be reduced to allow vertical development of the incisors and to establish incisor contact.

RADIAL CONSIDERATIONS

The buccal extension of the labial bow serves to reduce the pressure on the buccal aspect of the teeth and this, coupled with the facility to add cold-cure acrylic on the palatal aspect of the appliance, enables crossbite correction to be achieved.

The appliance is not suitable for use in crowded cases and is not amenable to simultaneous use with other appliances.

Management of the appliance

Adequate impressions are required and the working postured relationship is recorded with the incisors in an edge-to-edge position; if it is not possible for the patient to achieve this position, an intermediate posture can be used but it may be preferable in this situation to consider an alternative appliance.

FITTING THE APPLIANCE

The absence of any lingual extensions and palatal acrylic makes fitting the appliance simple. Initially the appliance is fitted in the untrimmed state. Patients very quickly tolerate the appliance because of its small bulk and should be expected to wear it at school within 2 weeks of first fitting the appliance.

ADJUSTMENT AND ACTIVATION

Trimming of the facets on the bionator are similar to the trimming of an Andresen appliance, except for the retention of an acrylic shelf similar to the occlusal shelf of the activator. Because of the design of the appliance this shelf only extends half-way across the occlusal surface of the posterior teeth. Progressive reduction of this shelf is carried out, usually of the molars first followed by trimming in the premolar region. When necessary, cold-cure acrylic may be added to inhibit vertical development of groups of teeth. The interdental spurs of acrylic are kept to help develop the intermaxillary force. Some operators prefer to design the appliance with acrylic contact only on the palatal and lingual aspect of the posterior teeth, and avoid the need for chairside trimming.

When using the appliance during the mixed dentition, loss of deciduous teeth tends to impair the fit of the appliance. The appliance cannot be reactivated and therefore a second appliance has to be made if reactivation is required.

The retention phase usually requires the removal of all the occlusal shelves to allow full intercuspation of the posterior teeth and a reduction in the hours of wear.

Reference

Ellisdon, P. & Hunt, N. (1985) The bionator: its use and abuse. *Dental Update*, **51**, 129.

Further reading

Eirew, H.L. (1981) The bionator. *British Journal of Orthodontics*, **8**, 33.
Heig, D.G.O., Callaert, H. & Opdebeek, H.M. (1989) The effect of the amount of protrusion built into the bionator. *American Journal of Orthodontics*, **95**, 401.

The function regulator

The function regulator of Frankel is a flexible appliance, the design of which is based upon rather different principles to the rigid acrylic functional appliance. Its originator claims that it is an exercise appliance, and that by retraining the facial muscles and the muscles of mastication to occupy new positions, the mandible and maxilla will be influenced to grow into corrected positions.

Design of the appliance

The appliance differs from other functional appliances mainly in that it incorporates thin acrylic shields which extend into the buccal sulci. The function of these is to hold the cheeks away from the teeth and alveolus to encourage the development of new bone, in either the maxillary or the mandibular arch. The shields are intended to apply tension on the underlying periosteum, encouraging new bone apposition. In addition, by holding the buccal tissues away from the alveolus, the shields also allow the action

of the tongue to expand the arches. This 'natural expansion' is claimed to be more beneficial than expansion achieved by mechanical means since it is said to be more stable.

There are three main types of the appliance which incorporate a variety of modifications. They are known by the initials FR1, FR2 and FR3. The appliances which are in common use are the FR1, for the treatment of Class II division 1 malocclusions (Fig. 6.14), and the FR3, for the treatment of Class III malocclusions. The FR2 is used for the treatment of Class II division 2 malocclusion and by some for Class II division 1 malocclusions. These appliances will be described in this text. The basic components of the function regulator are as follows:

1 Buccal shields

These remove muscle pressure from the outer aspects of the buccal segment teeth, and also extend into the sulcus, where they are designed to stretch the mucosa periosteum. They are also partly responsible for maintaining the vertical position of the mandible. The periphery of the shields is rounded and polished; the shields are of uniform thickness and are not in contact with the buccal surfaces of the teeth, or the alveolus (Fig. 6.15).

2 Lip pads

These are positioned in the labial sulcus and hold the lip away from the alveolus (Fig. 6.16). In the FR1 and FR2 they are positioned in the lower sulcus, to allow forward development of the mandibular alveolar process. In a Class III case they are placed in the maxillary sulcus with the aim of encouraging the development of maxillary alveolar bone.

3 Labial arch

This contacts the incisors with the aim of restricting their vertical development. The labial arch is passive unless the incisors are proclined and spaced, and require retraction. In a Class III case the labial arch is placed on the lower incisors.

4 Palatal arch

This connects the distal aspect of both buccal shields and passes deep in the embrasure mesial to the first molars, and across the

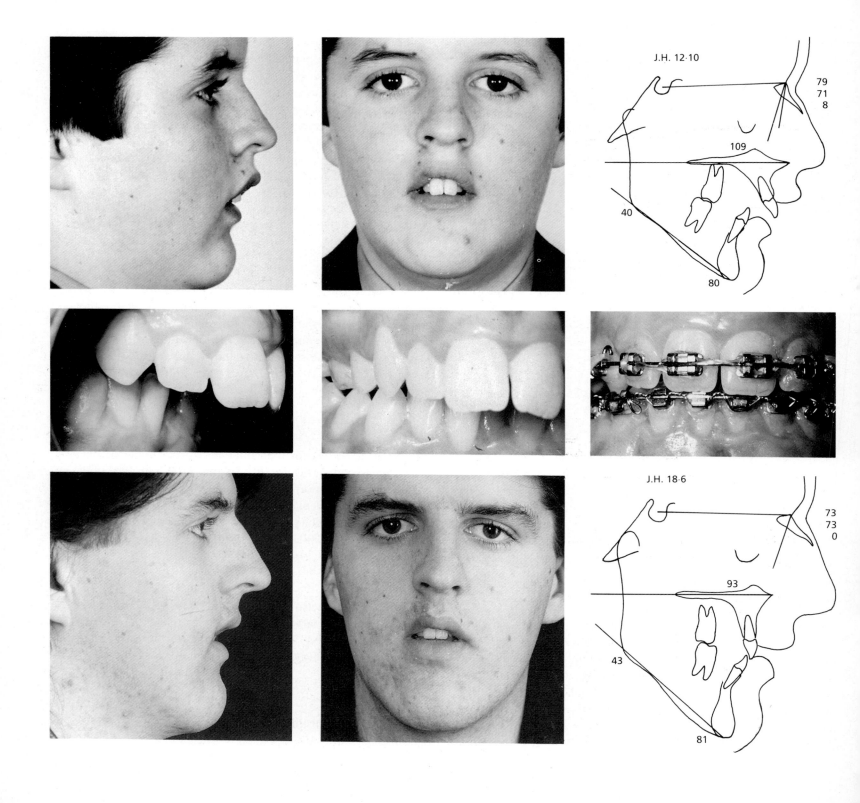

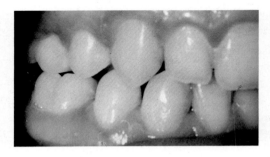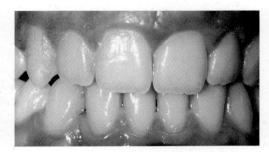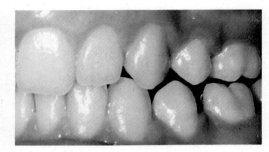

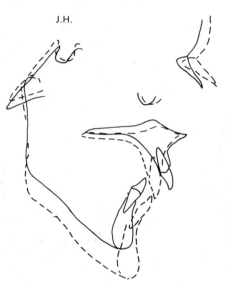

Fig. 6.14 J.H.: A Class II division 1 malocclusion with an overjet of 15 mm treated with an FR1 to reduce the skeletal discrepancy. Treatment was completed with second premolar extractions, fixed appliance and light headgear support.

palate, but does not contact the palatal mucosa. The ends of the palatal arch re-emerge from the buccal shields, and form occlusal stops on the first molars. These restrict vertical and forward development of the molars.

5 Lingual pads or wire

These are positioned lingual to the lower alveolus, and in conjunction with the lower labial pads encourage the forward posture of the mandible, by contacting the lingual mucosa and reminding the patient to hold the mandible in its new functional position.

6 Canine clasps

These pass from the buccal shields distal to the canine and should be firmly in contact with the mesial aspect of the first premolar or first deciduous molar. The anterior end is recurved on to the buccal surface of the canine.

Principal modifications

FR3

In the FR3, the lip pads are in the maxillary sulcus (Fig. 6.17), and the labial arch is in contact with the lower incisors. There is an anterior palatal arch which contacts the palatal aspect of the upper incisors to aid proclination of these teeth and this has an occlusal extension in contact with the lower molars to restrict vertical and forward development. The canine clasps and the lower lingual pads are omitted as there is no need to stimulate bone apposition on the anterior aspect of the mandible.

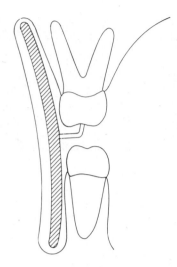

Fig. 6.15 Buccal shields—a cross-sectional view to show the relationship of the shield to the alveolar mucosa and buccal sulcus.

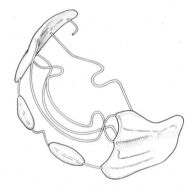

Fig. 6.16 Lip pads and labial arch.

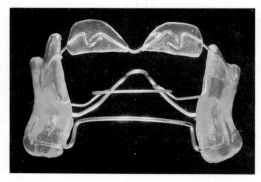

Fig. 6.17 FR3 appliance.

FR2

In the FR2, which is used for the management of Class II division 2 occlusions and by many for the treatment of Class II division 1 occlusions (instead of the FR1) there is an anterior palatal arch contacting the central incisors, which can be adjusted to procline these teeth. The canine clasps contact the buccal surfaces of the canines only.

Indications for the appliance

The appliance's main advantage is that its small bulk makes it easy for the patient to tolerate, and it is possible to achieve full-time wear, with the exception of eating. Normal speech with the appliance is also relatively easy to accomplish. Its rather fragile construction renders it very liable to distortion and adjustments to correct this can be difficult, time-consuming and sometimes impossible.

The treatment of Class II division 1 malocclusions is carried out with the FR1. It is a suitable appliance for the management of such occlusions and it is popular because it is readily accepted. The tendency for the lower labial segment to become proclined during treatment is more marked with a Frankel appliance and there is evidence (Robertson 1983) that more dento-alveolar change occurs when using the Frankel appliance than with other functional appliances. The Class II division 1 case with an everted lower lip trapped behind the upper labial segment is an ideal case to treat with a Frankel because the lower lip pads advance and unfurl the lower lip during treatment bringing it in front of the upper incisors. This feature not only speeds upper incisor retraction but also produces an immediate improvement in the patient's facial appearance. Recent work has shown that the functional regulator gives an improved facial profile (Battagel 1987) and that there is less root resorption of the incisor apices (Hawthorn 1987) compared with cases treated with headgear and fixed appliances. When treating Class II division 2 malocclusions it is possible to follow the same regimen as for the activator and to convert the incisor occlusion into Class II division 1 form with an upper removable appliance and then correct the underlying discrepancy to Class I using a Frankel appliance. However, it is also possible in a mild case to carry out the upper arch alignment using the FR2 alone by a simple modification of the palatal aspect of the appliance. Palatal wires engage the central incisors and procline these whilst the Frankel corrects the antero-posterior relationship. In many Class II division 2 malocclusions it is acceptable to allow a certain amount of lower labial segment proclination in the knowledge that this is likely to remain stable after treatment. It is also possible to accept some mild lower arch crowding at the completion of treatment. The management of excessive traumatic overbites in established Class II division 2 malocclusions is not recommended with the function regulator alone, simply because the degree of vertical skeletal discrepancy in such cases is usually beyond the scope of functional appliances, the Frankel included. If treatment can be started in the mixed dentition however, the use of an FR2 can encourage proclination of the lower labial segment, which may prevent the development of an excessive overbite.

To date, the FR3 appliance is the best functional appliance to use in the management of Class III occlusions (Fig. 6.18). The amount of change in a true skeletal discrepancy that can be achieved is limited but the Frankel appliance may offer a greater change than is possible with fixed appliances alone. Many clinicians use the FR3 appliance in Class III cases where there is a postural or displacing activity of the mandible. The authors prefer to treat such occlusions by simpler means — removable appliances from choice — to enable correction of the displacing activity and simultaneous proclination of the upper labial segment. The authors find the FR3 suitable in those cases where there is no displacement of the mandible, a reduced overbite and little prospect of correcting the incisor relationship by upper arch proclination alone. The amount of correction that can be achieved is, of course, limited, and marked or severe Class 3 skeletal patterns can only be corrected surgically. Similarly, the long-term prognosis for cases that have been corrected with functional appliances must be guarded in view of the tendency for mandibular growth to continue during late adolescence, especially in boys.

VERTICAL CONTROL AND RADIAL CHANGES

In situations where the overbite is excessive, the Frankel appliance is of limited use. This is because the appliance does not directly control the upper or lower incisor vertical position, unlike the more rigid appliances. Overbite correction with the Frankel appliance mostly depends upon natural adjustment of the buccal segments once the incisor relationship has been corrected.

In the management of anterior openbites, a specific appliance design is recommended. Frankel & Frankel (1983) show several cases which have been managed with such an appliance but the majority of these are in the younger age group where secondary factors are often playing an important part in the maintenance of the anterior openbite. The authors have had no success in the use of a Frankel appliance in a true skeletal openbite case.

Buccal crossbite correction during management of a Class II division 1 malocclusion is easy with a function regulator as the appliance places the mandible in a postured position with both condyles symmetrically placed thus eliminating any displacement. The buccal shields encourage upper arch expansion.

Where there is a lingual crossbite it is necessary to take a sufficiently high bite registration to ensure that the expansion of the lower arch is not inhibited by the occlusion. The buccal shields in such a case are well relieved away from the alveolus in the lower arch with minimal relief in the upper arch.

Mixed dentition cases are ideally treated with the Frankel appliance. The authors, however, except in extreme cases, prefer not to institute treatment before the age of 10 years. This is because they consider that the majority of children in the United Kingdom are not sufficiently mature or motivated to manage the appliances any earlier. Also, early commencement of treatment considerably lengthens the overall treatment time. The appliance is suitable in the mixed dentition because of the absence of any close-fitting components that contact the teeth. The change from the mixed to the permanent dentition can thus take place without the need for a new appliance. Frankel suggests that the wire from the buccal shield which crosses the occlusal surfaces of the posterior teeth and the palate should engage a prepared notch cut in the second upper deciduous molars. A spirited correspondence between Frankel and others on the relative merits of such discing is reported in the *Americal Journal of Orthodontics* (1984) and deserves attention.

Although many use the appliance in crowded cases and claim that this overcomes the need for extractions, the authors take the conservative view that the use of functional appliances to achieve upper arch expansion is not a guaranteed way to relieve crowding in the long term. The selection of those crowded cases which will not relapse following expansion with appliances is difficult. The natural tendency when using the Frankel appliance is for expansion of both upper and lower arches to occur.

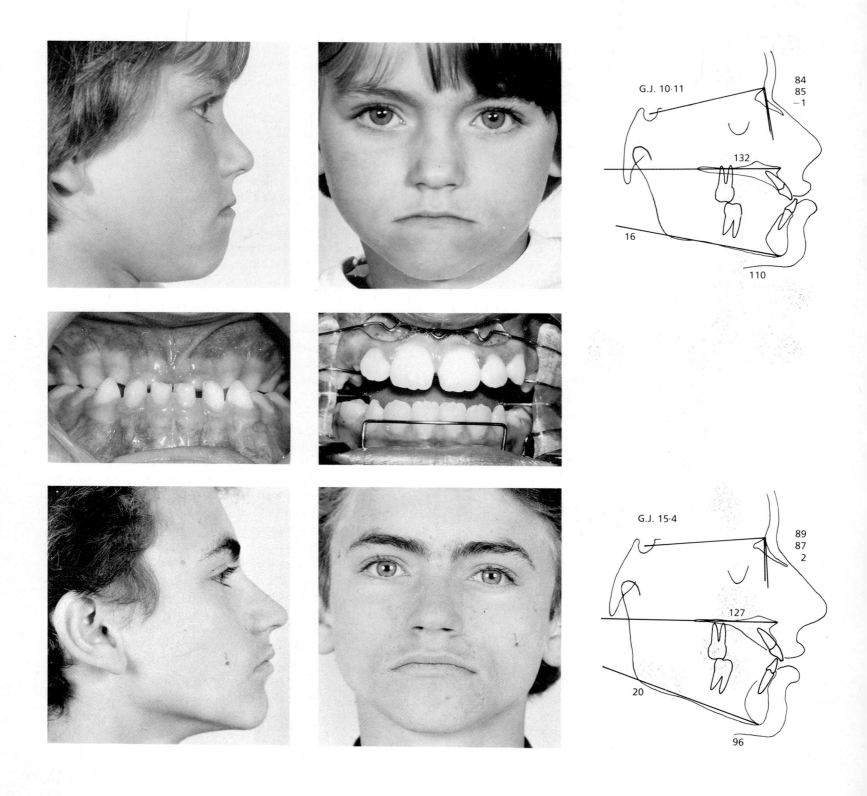

G.J. 10·11

84
85
−1

132

16

110

G.J. 15·4

89
87
2

127

20

96

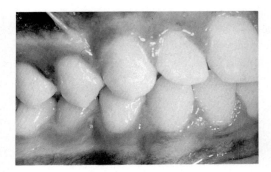 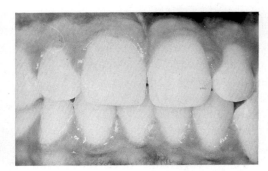 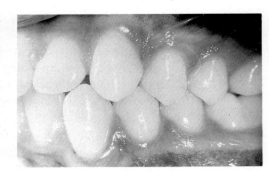

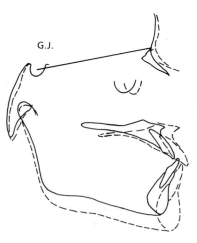

Fig. 6.18 G.J.: Although referred originally in the deciduous dentition, treatment was not started until the age of 11 years. The reversed overjet was 2 mm and there was no displacing activity of the mandible. The occlusion was corrected with an FR3 appliance alone and is shown 4 years out of retention.

Management of the appliance

Impressions must be taken specifically for the construction of this appliance. Trays with reasonably extended flanges should be used, and tray edging wax added both to aid retention of the impression material and to ensure that the impression is adequately extended into the buccal sulcus. It is essential to try the tray in the mouth with the peripheral wax in position before taking the impression and to mould the wax into the reflection of the sulcus.

The occlusal registration is made by opening the mandible to just beyond the freeway space. The mandible is postured forwards and care must be taken to avoid any lateral shift. In a Class II division 1 case the mandible is brought forward to approximately half the distance of its possible maximum protrusion. In Class III cases the mandible is simply held in a partially open position, but with slightly wider opening than is used for a Class II case.

Fitting must be undertaken with care as the appliance is easily distorted and once distorted is extremely difficult to correct. As always it is helpful to show the patient the appliance first. The appliance is best inserted by placing one side in the mouth then rotating the appliance round fully into the mouth. The patient practises this in a mirror, then demonstrates it to the parent. The appliance should be checked to ensure that the periphery of the buccal shields extends into the reflection of the mucosa without impinging directly onto the alveolar mucosa. It is important to explain that care must be taken in handling the appliance and to provide a rigid container in which to keep it when not in wear.

As has been said earlier, Frankel uses the appliance as an exercise appliance. He recommends a very gradual increase in the number of hours during which the appliance is worn. The authors' preference is to use the standard routine of 6 hours a day training for two weeks followed by a check appointment, when any necessary adjustments can be made prior to the patient wearing the appliance full-time (except for eating and sport).

The appliance is invariably tolerated extremely well and speech should closely approach normal after a week or two. The patients are instructed to keep their lips together at all times, and to carry out lip seal exercises when they are doing their homework or watching television. This involves pressing their lips together and contracting them against the appliance. The forward posture that is induced by wearing the appliance offers an immediate improvement in the profile, although the bulk of the labial shield tends to give the patient a slightly chubby appearance.

MANAGEMENT OF THE OCCLUSION

In addition to the routine measurement of the overjet and assessment of the molar relationship at each visit, the intercanine distance and intermolar width should be monitored. An excessive increase in intercanine width, particularly in the lower arch, should, in the authors' view, be avoided. A clinical estimation of the lower labial segment inclination can be made, and should this appear to be proclining, then a cephalometric radiograph is essential. If excessive proclination has occurred, it may be necessary to overtreat the case, bearing in mind that the lower incisor angulation will return at least partially to its original position after the completion of treatment thereby causing some relapse in the overjet (Mills 1968).

A certain amount of adjustment of the appliance can be made by bending the various wire components:

1   A limited amount of adjustment of the support wires is possible to ensure that the labial pads are correctly positioned in the sulcus.

2   Very light activation of the trans-palatal arch may be necessary to ensure that the buccal shields are out of contact with the buccal surface of the teeth and the buccal alveolar mucosa.

3   The canine clasps may require adjustment to allow full eruption of the canines, for example to ensure that the acrylic shields are out of contact.

The labial arch is not designed to close incisor spacing and must not be activated to apply a force to the incisors. Provided the appliance has been correctly made and an accurate impression of the vestibular sulcus has been obtained, it is not usually necessary to trim the acrylic at the periphery of the vestibular shields.

The whole appliance can be reactivated by repositioning the labial pads, which should be carried out when the overjet reduction has rendered the mandibular posture ineffective. This is achieved by drilling through the buccal acrylic shield to release the wire carrying the pads. The pad is advanced and the wire held in its new position by the addition of cold-cure acrylic (Fig. 6.19).

DETAILING AND RETENTION

It is not possible to utilize fixed appliances concurrently with Frankel appliances, or to use headgear simultaneously. When necessary, fixed appliance treatment is usually carried out subsequent to initial sagittal correction with a Frankel appliance.

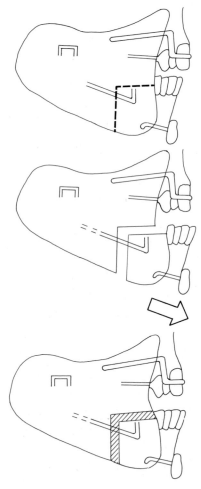

Fig. 6.19 Reactivation — the wire carrying the lip pads is released and the buccal shields advanced into the new position.

The appliance does not require any modification to enter a retention period. All that is required is for it to be worn for a reduced period of time. If this is the sole method of treatment, it may be necessary to maintain part time wear until the maximum pubertal growth spurt has passed.

References

Battagel, J. (1989) Profile changes in Class II division 1 malocclusions: A comparison of the effects of Edgewise and Frankel therapy. *European Journal of Orthodontics*, **11**, 243.

Frankel, R. (1984) Correspondence. *American Journal of Orthodontics*, **85**, 441.

Frankel, R. & Frankel, C. (1983) A functional approach to treatment of skeletal open bite. *American Journal of Orthodontics*, **84**, 63.

Hawthorn, I.S. (1987) MSc Report (abstract), *British Journal of Orthodontics*, **14**, 313.

Robertson N.R.E. (1983). Treatment changes in children treated with the function regulator. *American Journal of Orthodontics*, **83**, 299.

Further reading

Creekmore, T.D. & Radney, L.J. (1983) Frankel appliance therapy. *American Journal of Orthodontics*, **83**, 89.

Eirew, H.L., McDowell, F. & Phillips, J.G. (1976) The FR3. *British Journal of Orthodontics*, **3**, 67.

Falck, F. & Frankel, R. (1989) Step by step mandibular advancement in the treatment of mandibular retrusion using the Frankel appliance. *American Journal of Orthodontics*, **96**, 333.

Frankel, R. (1980) A functional approach to oro-facial orthopaedics. *British Journal of Orthodontics*, **7**, 41.

Gianelly, A.A., Arena, S.A. & Bernsein, L. (1984) A comparison of Class II treatment changes noted with straight wire, edgewise and Frankel appliance. *American Journal of Orthodontics*, **86**, 269.

Loh, N.K. & Kerr, W.J.S. (1985) The FR3. Effects and indications. *British Journal of Orthodontics*, **12**, 153.

McDougall, P.D., McNamara, J.A. Jr & Dierkes, J.M. (1982) Arch width in Class II patients treated with Functional Regulator. *American Journal of Orthondontics*, **82**, 10.

McNamara, J.A. Jr & Huge, S.A. (1981) The FR2. *American Journal of Orthodontics*, **80**, 478.

McNamara, J.A. Jr & Huge, S.A. (1985) The FR3. *American Journal of Orthodontics*, **88**, 409.

Nielsen, I.L. (1984) Facial growth during treatment with Functional Regulator. *American Journal of Orthodontics*, **85**, 401.

Remmer, K.R., Mamandras, A.H. & Way, D.C. (1985) Cephalometric changes associated with Activator, FR, and fixed appliance. *American Journal of Orthodontics*, **88**, 363.

The twin block

This appliance is a unique, ingenious appliance which, unlike any other functional appliance so far described, is formed and worn

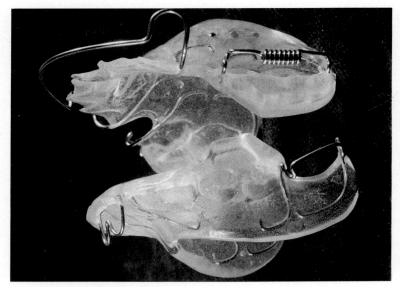

Fig. 6.20 Twin block appliance.

in two parts. These carry inclined planes which meet and cause the mandible to be postured forwards on closure (Fig. 6.20). The appliance is well tolerated and it may easily be worn full-time. The maxillary appliance incorporates attachments for headgear. The mandibular appliance carries a hook to attach an elastic to the headgear facebow.

Headgear may be attached to the upper part of the appliance by means of a face bow which engages coils incorporated on modified Adams clasps. The appliance can be used satisfactorily in the mixed dentition but may require remaking when a number of deciduous teeth have been shed.

In cases that exhibit crowding and rotations or marked displacement of teeth, the appliance is not suitable as the close fit of the acrylic to the occlusal surfaces prevents any individual tooth movement. Similarly, cases where extractions are carried out, and some spontaneous alignment is to take place during the functional stage of treatment, cannot easily be managed with this appliance.

Design of the appliance

The upper part of the appliance is similar to a removable appliance with molar capping. The molar capping is limited to the posterior end of the arch with an inclined plane at the mesial end. This plane engages a similar incline on the lower appliance and causes the mandible to be postured forwards (Fig. 6.21). A midline screw is incorporated to provide compensatory upper arch expansion as the antero-posterior relationship improves. The clasps used for retention are modified Adams which span the second premolars and first molars. The bridge of the Adams clasp is wound in a short coil and this enables a headgear face bow to be added without the usual weakness associated with soldered tubes (Fig. 6.22). An anterior U-loop labial bow (0.7 mm) is incorporated. The lower part of the appliance carries capping in the premolar region only. The lower section is retained by Adams clasps and 'C' clasps on the canines — anterior retention is designed to reduce proclination of the lower labial segment and may be by clasps or, in the authors' hands, by acrylic covering the incisor tips and about one-third of the labial aspect of the incisors. Some lingual extension also helps to distribute the mesially directed forces on to the mandibular alveolus as distinct from the mandibular teeth.

In its original form as described by Clark (1982), the lower section incorporates a hook which is connected by elastics to the extra-oral face bow. The purpose of this is to encourage forward posture of the mandible. In common with many other users, we omit this as it has been found to be an effective appliance without this additional complication.

Clinical considerations

In the management of a Class II division 1 malocclusion, the twin block appliance is excellent, because it can be worn continuously, progress is good and occasionally rapid. Class II division 2 malocclusions can also be managed provided that the lower arch is well aligned and free of crowding. Because the upper part of the appliance is retained firmly by means of clasps, springs to procline the central incisors can be incorporated. A separate course of treatment to convert the incisor relationship into Class II division 1 is not required. A Class III version of the appliance is described; however this does not appear to have any clear advantage over conventional appliances.

VERTICAL CONSIDERATIONS

In the management of increased overbite, the twin block appliance is not as efficient as the activator as there is less opportunity to allow unimpeded vertical growth of the posterior teeth. Its use in low maxillary—mandibular plane angle cases is therefore not indicated.

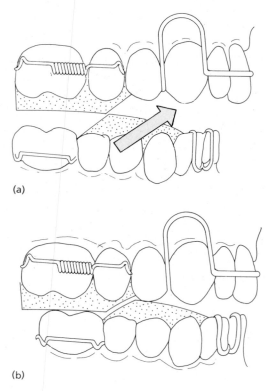

(a)

(b)

Fig. 6.21 The action of the inclined planes is to posture the mandible forwards.

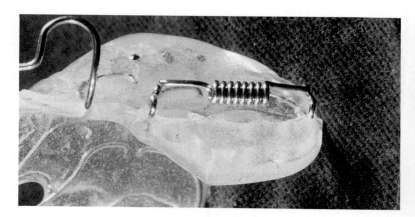

Fig. 6.22 An extended Adams clasp incorporating a coil to accommodate a face bow.

RADIAL CONSIDERATIONS

Because the appliance incorporates a screw, it is satisfactory in the management of patients who have a crossbite. It may also be used in the more uncommon circumstances where there is a buccal crossbite or boxbite. The upper appliance then incorporates a screw in the open position which is closed during treatment. The occlusal coverage enables the occlusion to be unlocked and the advancement of the mandible brings a wider part of the mandible into a better relationship with the maxillary teeth.

Management of the appliance

Adequate impressions with good lower lingual extensions are required, and the working postural relationship is taken with the mandible in protrusion with sufficient opening to allow for a total of 5 mm thickness of molar covering. Care should be taken not to protrude the mandible more than about half the amount of total protrusion that is possible as reactivation once the appliance is worn is easily achieved.

FITTING THE APPLIANCE

Both parts of the appliance must be fitted at the same time, but the fitting of the headgear may be delayed until after the intra-oral appliance is accepted. As with other appliances, a 2-week training period is recommended, with 6 hours a day wear, followed by a check appointment and then progression to full-time wear. Eating with the appliance is difficult but many patients can manage this. For those who can, it is wise to point out the need to clean the appliance and teeth carefully afterwards as the molar capping can give rise to food stagnation.

The extra-oral appliance is fitted at the second or third visit using a standard U-loop face bow and full headgear. The amount of wear required depends on the severity of the malocclusion but 14 hours a day wear is an average target. In mild cases, headgear may not be required at all.

ADJUSTMENT AND ACTIVATION

The retention of the appliance is good and clasps require only occasional adjustment simply to maintain adequate retention. The longer clasp on the upper premolar and molar incorporating the coil for the headgear is more flexible than a conventional Adams clasp, but this does not give rise to problems. The rigid clasping eliminates the possibility of passive expansion. Thus regular adjustment of the upper midline screw is required to prevent a crossbite from developing as the antero-posterior relationship is correcting. The screw requires activation of about a quarter turn a month, unless there is also an existing crossbite which requires correction. It is often sufficient for the operator to undertake screw adjustment at the time of the regular monthly visit. Treatment progress must be checked regularly and care taken to ensure that an apparent reduction in overjet is not due to a false posture. A lateral openbite is likely to develop as the effect of the inhibition of vertical development on the buccal segments takes place, and also as the overjet reduces. Reactivation of the postural element is by the addition of cold-cure acrylic to the inclined planes. This is usually most conveniently achieved in the mouth by the addition of cold cure to the lower appliance. The molar capping of the upper appliance should be covered with petroleum jelly to prevent adhesion between the two halves (Fig. 6.23).

During correction of the antero-posterior relationship the molar occlusion is allowed to re-establish by progressive reduction of the upper molar block (Fig. 6.24). Eventually the lower appliance can be discarded to allow full buccal intercuspation to establish, and the upper appliance can be kept as a retainer maintaining headgear support if necessary (Fig. 6.25).

COMBINATION TREATMENT

Apart from the fact that headgear is used with the appliance, it is not suitable to use this functional appliance technique simul-

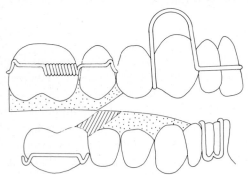

Fig. 6.23 Reactivation of a twin block appliance.

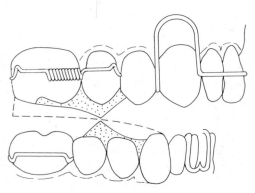

Fig. 6.24 The method of trimming the upper molar covering during treatment.

taneously with full arch fixed attachments. If fixed appliances are used, they must be fitted at the completion of the functional stage of the treatment. Only segmental labial fixed appliances can be used during the functional phase of treatment. These can be converted to full arch appliances once the twin block appliance is discarded.

Reference

Clark, W.J. (1982) The Twin Block traction technique. *European Journal of Orthodontics*, **4**, 129.

Further reading

Clark, W.J. (1988) The Twin Block technique. *American Journal of Orthodontics*, **3**, 1.
Trenouth, M.J. (1989) A functional appliance system for the correction of Class II relationships. *British Journal of Orthodontics*, **16**, 169.

Notes on other appliances

Oral screen

This is a forerunner of the functional regulator appliance and consists of a vestibular shield which holds the lips away from the buccal aspect of all the teeth with the exception of the upper incisors, which are left in contact with the appliance. The pressure from the lips is transferred to the upper incisors and acts to move them palatally. One of the advantages of the appliance is that it can be used in the mixed dentition and also that it aids patients with digit-sucking habits. It is little used now following reports of possible exessive apical resorption.

Positioners

These devices are usually used as retaining appliances following fixed appliance treatment, are made of flexible plastic and carry impressions of the upper and lower dental arches. They are made into a slightly overtreated Class I relationship. The patient wears the positioner immediately following band removal and is taught to clench the teeth into the positioner. The action is a combination of moulding the individual teeth into their correct positions within the arches by the effect of the plastic in contact with the teeth, but it also has a functional element of establishing a correct inter-arch relationship. The appliances are available commercially in a range of different sizes, but to obtain the best results custom-made positioners are the most effective. These are constructed from up-to-date models. The individual teeth are cut from the model and set up in an ideal relationship before the positioner is constructed. Whilst having the advantage of retaining upper and lower arches at the same time as normal function takes place, the amount of antero-posterior change possible with such appliance is limited.

The Bimler appliance

There are three main kinds of Bimler appliance: type A for Class II division 1 occlusion, type B for Class II division 2 malocclusion and type C for Class III occlusion.

These are flexible appliances and carry labial and lingual springs and bows in both arches connected together by two acrylic wings which just engage the palatal mucosa. Each appliance type is further subdivided into two main categories, space creation or space closure, the space creation variety carrying additional active springs.

The type A appliance has a preformed labial splint on the labial aspect of the lower incisors and springs on the lingual aspect of the lower incisors, the mandible being held in its postured position by the incisors engaging this splint. There is a lower labial wire which holds the splint in position and connects distally with the acrylic, thereby to the upper part of the appliance. The upper part of the appliance carries a labial arch and palatal spring. The two acrylic springs are connected by a coffin spring.

The type B appliance has acrylic palatal coverage, with a midline screw, and there is no labial arch on the upper incisors.

The type C appliance has occlusal wires covered with plastic

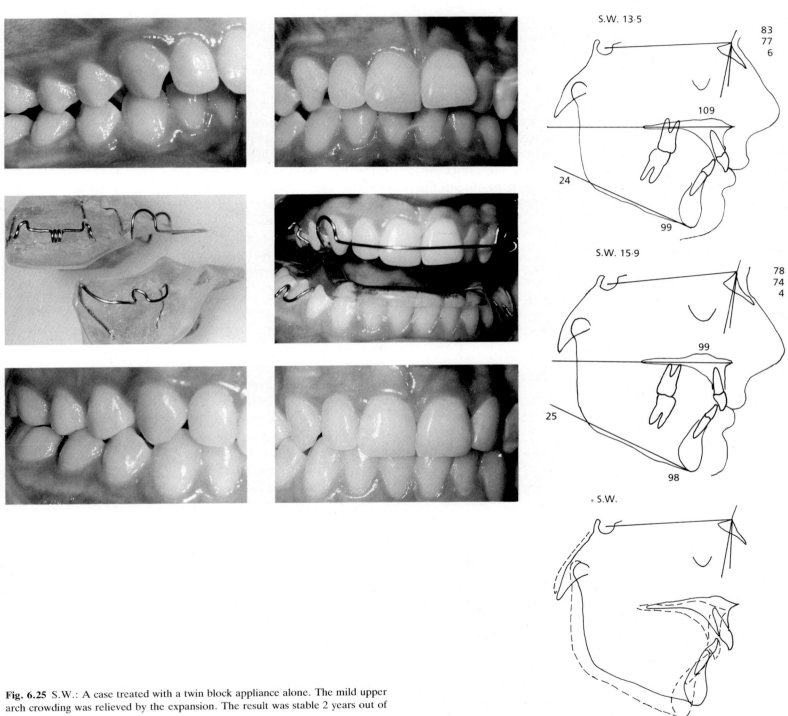

Fig. 6.25 S.W.: A case treated with a twin block appliance alone. The mild upper arch crowding was relieved by the expansion. The result was stable 2 years out of retention.

tubing to achieve bite opening. There is no labial splint, but the lower incisors are retracted by a labial bow originating from the upper part of the appliance.

The Herbst appliance

This appliance is a fixed functional appliance, completely tooth-borne. It is cemented to the arches and is permanently connected by a telescopic spring device which postures the mandible forwards. In its original form cast metal skeleton splints are cemented to both upper and lower arches and once placed by the operator cannot be removed by the patient (Fig. 6.26).

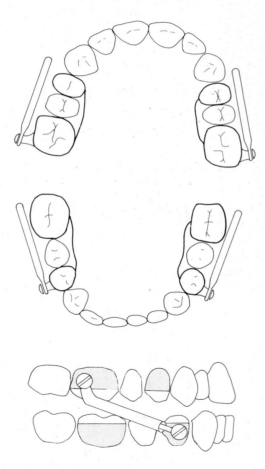

Fig. 6.26 Herbst appliance. Rods fixed to the lower arch engage tubes which are attached to the upper molar bands and hold the mandible in forward posture.

As might be expected, because most of the force is delivered directly to the teeth, there is an increased tendency for lower incisor proclination to occur during treatment (Pancherz & Pancherz 1982) but because of the enforced full-time wear the occlusal changes are very rapid.

A more recent variation in this design is used by McNamara (1988) in which the coverage of the teeth is by means of acrylic splints. The upper splint is in two acrylic sections each extending from the canines to the back of the arch. They are connected by a hyrax expansion screw.

The lower splint has complete occlusal coverage. The upper and lower splints are coupled together by spring-loaded arms, as in the conventional appliance. Some operators use this appliance as a totally removable appliance, whilst others prefer to cement the upper part of the appliance to the arch by an acid etch technique, leaving only the lower splint removable by the patient.

Lip bumper

This appliance which can be used in both the maxilla and mandible uses the muscular force from the upper or lower lip to provide a distal force, usually to the first molars. The appliance has something in common with the labial pads on the FR appliances which also displace the lip forwards and perhaps downwards. There is little inclination to use lip bumpers in the upper arch as most orthodontists would find a face bow and headgear force simpler and more effective although Salzman (1957) suggested its use as an adjunct to headgear force.

In the lower arch, however, headgear is much less acceptable and so a lip bumper can be useful. The appliance has two effects. Firstly by removing the soft tissue forces from the labial aspect of the lower anteriors it may produce forward tilting of these teeth under the influence of the tongue. This tooth movement may be undesirable but can be reduced by siting the bumper as low as possible in the labial sulcus so that the upper part of the lip is able to maintain contact with the incisors. This unwanted effect can also be controlled if the lower anterior teeth are banded. The desired and therapeutic second effect of the lip bumper is to move the anchor teeth distally (usually first molars). The degree of distal movement can be very limited, especially where the second molars are erupted. Such distal movement is most effective when lower second molars have been extracted, usually in an arch where only a small amount of distal movement of the first molars is required to relieve anterior crowding.

Application of the lip bumper, which may be custom-made in the laboratory or obtained ready-made in several sizes, is to tubes on the molar teeth. In the upper arch where headgear tubes are often standard features of the buccal assemblies this is relatively easy to do. In the lower, unless a further set of special molar bands are held in stock, round tubes will need to be added to the bands. This is not always a convenient exercise in the surgery. The extra tubes can also often interfere with the occlusion.

References

McNamara, J.A. Jr (1988) Fabrication of the acrylic splint Herbst appliance. *American Journal of Orthodontics*, **94**, 10.

Pancherz, A. & Pancherz, M. (1982) Bite jumping with the Herbst appliance. *European Journal of Orthodontics*, **4**, 37.

Salzman, J.A. (1957) *Orthodontics, Practice and Techniques*, p. 328. Lippincott, Philadelphia.

Further reading

Bimler, H.P. (1985) The Bimler appliance. *Journal of Clinical Orthodontics*, **19**, 880.

Dixon, D.A. (1958) Vestibular anchorage; a clinical experiment. *Transactions of the British Society for the Study of Orthodontics*, **45**, 100.

Howe, R.P. (1987) Removable plastic Herbst treatment. *American Journal of Orthodontics*, **92**, 275.

Mischler, W.A. & Delivinas, H.P. (1984) A comparison study between three tooth positioners. *American Journal of Orthodontics*, **85**, 154.

Owman-Moll, P. & Ingervall, B. (1984) Effects of oral screen treatment. *American Journal of Orthodontics*, **85**, 37.

Wieslander, L. (1984) Intensive treatment of severe Class II malocclusions with a Headgear−Herbst appliance in the early mixed dentition. *American Journal of Orthodontics*, **86**, 1.

Chapter 7

The Use of Functional Appliances with Other Forms of Treatment

In combination with other appliances

As Harvold pointed out, functional appliances are nowadays seen to be essentially interceptive devices providing a useful part of the armamentarium of an orthodontist. A functional appliance will seldom provide a complete solution to an occlusal problem. Treatment will usually include the use of other appliances (Broadbent 1987). Nowadays functional appliances are frequently used in conjunction with headgear, lip bumpers, fixed appliances, and with maxillary removable appliances.

Due to the interceptive nature of functional appliances and because their use does not depend on the erupted presence of premolars and canines, most other forms of treatment will tend to follow the use of a functional appliance rather than precede it. However, on occasion they can be used concurrently and this is particularly true of headgear. With today's clinical standards it is now usual to complete most functional appliance cases with fixed appliances.

Removable appliances

Removable appliances play a small part in association with functional appliance therapy. Removable appliances have been used for some simple auxilliary tooth movements and in the right circumstances can be most useful. Some local tooth movements can conveniently be carried out in this simple manner either preceding or following functional appliance wear (Fig. 7.1). They are particularly effective in dealing with local crossbites of anterior or posterior teeth. Some workers advocate the addition of springs to the functional appliance itself. In the authors' view the displacing effect of activator springs unduly complicates treatment and makes the appliance less acceptable to the patient. We therefore only occasionally incorporate springs in functional appliances.

A typical example would be in the treatment of Class II division 2 malocclusion where upper central incisors are best proclined by a removable appliance prior to functional appliance therapy. Such a removable appliance can be designed to give retention against the displacing forces of the springs required to push the central incisors forwards against the lip force. In these circum-

stances, springs on the functional appliance itself would tend to unseat the appliance and be less effective. Although a fixed appliance will advance and align the incisors, a removable appliance can often achieve this but has the additional benefit of a bite plane which will assist in overbite reduction.

Some practitioners choose to combine functional appliance treatment with simultaneous wear of a removable appliance and instruct the patient to interchange the wear of the appliances. This requires the removable appliance to be worn during the day and the functional appliance whilst at home and asleep. The purpose of this is to produce some initial tooth movement (for instance expansion) with a removable appliance, and then to maintain the movement with the daytime wear and to achieve sagittal correction using the functional appliance worn during evenings and nights. The authors' preference is to seek maximum wear of the functional appliance wherever possible and therefore to design this to maintain any tooth movement previously attained with removable appliances. There is no reason why a functional appliance worn for the greater part of the day should not satisfactorily retain active tooth movement of this kind.

Headgear

There is some evidence (Teuscher 1978) that the combination of headgear with functional appliances enhances the clinical effectiveness of the treatment. It may also prove beneficial in modifying the effect of the functional appliance so as to control the vertical position of the upper incisors. Headgear may be readily added to an Andresen or activator type of appliance and there are a number of ways by which this can be done. High-pull headgear can also be used to assist the retention of an appliance when a patient finds that it is persistently dislodged during sleep.

METHODS OF COMBINING HEADGEAR WITH FUNCTIONAL APPLIANCES

1 Bands on first molars

A face bow can be applied to 0.045-inch tubes on molar bands and the appliance constructed to fit over these. Because the extra-oral force is directed to the first molars the effect on the rest of the maxillary arch will depend on the fit of the appliance around these teeth. The activator for instance will allow some differential distal movement of the molars to take place which may be of benefit in the relief of mild mid-buccal segment crowding. Appliances such as the Andresen with closely fitting acrylic around the buccal teeth will tend to transmit the extra-oral force more generally to the maxillary teeth.

2 Face bow directly to the appliance

Whilst it is possible to construct appliances with an integral face bow, the provision of a detachable face bow enables the functional appliance to be worn independently, with the advantage that additional wear of the functional appliance can be achieved. Small tubes are available which can be incorporated into the acrylic of appliances and these are usually placed in the molar region, so that standard commercially available face bows can be fitted (Fig. 7.2). If the appliance incorporates molar clasps (for example the twin block), tubes may be soldered to these. Alternatively a coil may be constructed within the clasps to accept the face bow.

With both these methods the inhibiting effect of a functional appliance on the forward development of the maxilla can then be enhanced by the extra-oral force (Fig. 7.3).

3 J-hooks to the appliance

Headgear can be attached to the anterior part of some appliances. Those carrying a U-loop labial bow or a similar anterior bow can have spurs bent in them, or these can be soldered to them. High-pull headgear is usually used with this form of application as it is an effective way of enhancing the retention of an appliance. The disadvantage of this method is that it may make the bow contact the incisors and cause incisor retroclination.

With rigid acrylic appliances it is possible to attach the J-hooks to small wire hooks which are incorporated in the acrylic at the angles of the mouth. This ensures that the extra-oral force is directed to the whole of the appliance, and is more satisfactory than applying the headgear to the labial bow. However, because there is a small but significant risk of facial damage should the J-hooks be dislodged, the authors usually choose other methods of applying headgear.

Direction of force

When the extra-oral force is applied to a functional appliance any form of cervical traction or pull directed horizontally is inappropriate, as this is liable to dislodge the appliance. A full headgear, such as the Interlandi, or a high-pull headgear is essential. It is usually considered to be desirable to direct the force to a point just above the apices of the molars; this is to produce the maximum amount of maxillary inhibition. If extra-oral force is being used to enhance retention of the appliance, especially at night, then an upwards component of force is clearly indicated.

Fixed appliances

It is sometimes appropriate to use fixed appliances simultaneously with functional appliance therapy. Depending upon the precise design of the appliance it is usually possible to place bands on upper or lower first molars and brackets can then be bonded to certain of the other teeth. In this way headgear wear can be commenced as outlined above, and some minor tooth movements can be simultaneously undertaken to align the labial or buccal teeth. Fixed appliances can also provide some assistance with bite opening in particularly deep bite cases.

Fixed appliances are most commonly used to complete a course of functional appliance therapy. The chief indication for this phase of treatment is to complete arch alignment, root paralleling and where necessary space closure. The choice of a particular fixed appliance system can influence the choice of extractions which may be prescribed during or before this phase of treatment. Such treatment can be completed with various forms of fixed appliance, such as Begg or edgewise, according to the operator's preference.

When transferring from a period of functional appliance therapy to fixed appliance therapy in a Class II case it must be remembered that the restraining effect of the appliance on the maxilla will cease when the appliance is left out. It is necessary to continue this restraint soon after the start of the fixed appliance phase of treatment. With a Begg appliance it will be possible to replace this force with Class II elastic traction. With most edgewise techniques it will usually be necessary to change the arch wire several times before it is possible to start Class II elastic traction. It is wise therefore to institute or continue light extra-oral force during this phase.

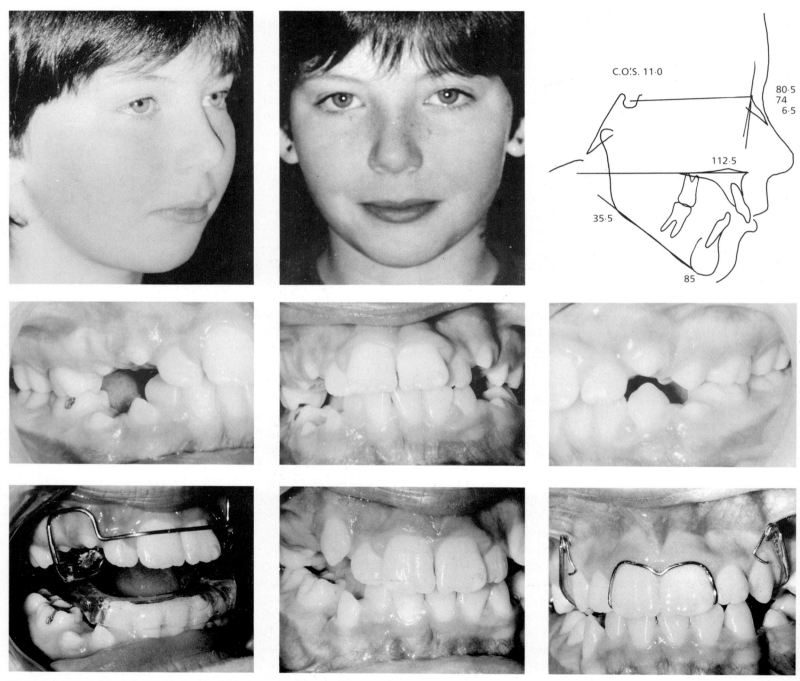

Fig. 7.1 C.O'S. A Class II division 1 malocclusion treated with an activator followed by a removable appliance. Four first premolars were extracted shortly after the activator was fitted.

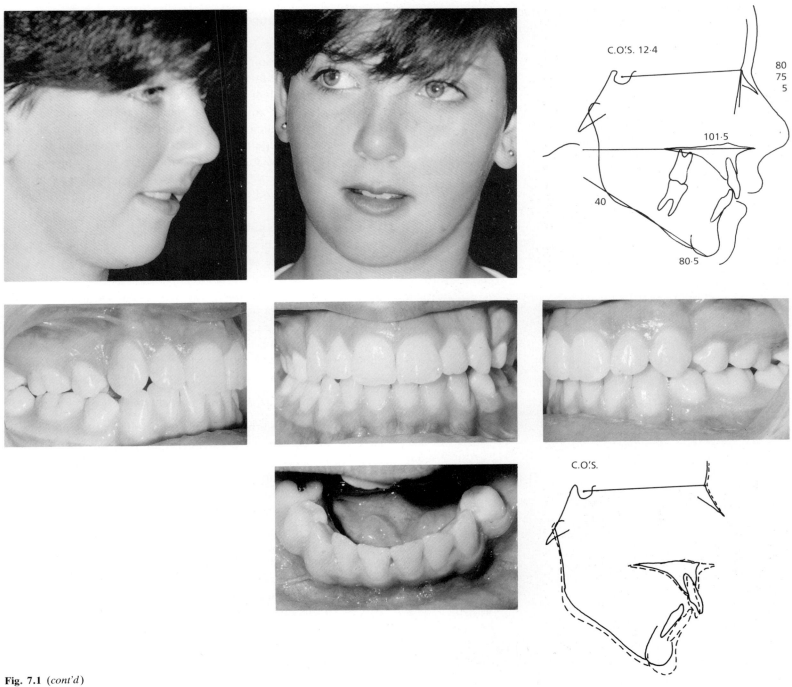

Fig. 7.1 (*cont'd*)

The principles of fixed appliance treatment after functional appliance therapy are otherwise no different from any other course of such treatment.

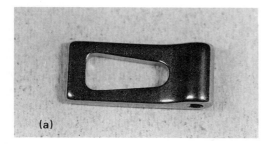

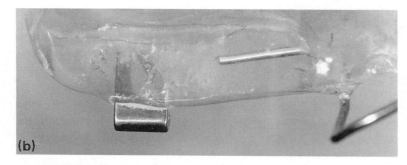

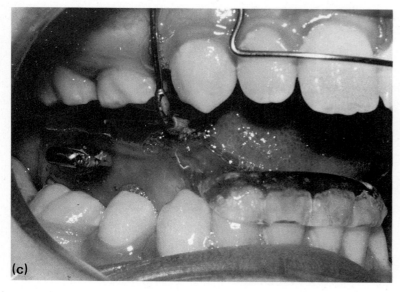

Fig. 7.2 Molar headgear tubes. (a) Cast chrome attachments; (b) incorporated into the acrylic of the occlusal shelf; (c) location in the mouth.

Functional appliances in combination with extractions

The traditional view is that functional appliances are essentially appropriate to the so-called 'non-extraction' group of cases, and is particularly associated with the Andresen appliance. Nevertheless the current view of combining extraction with functional treatment allows a considerable increase in the scope of cases treated and many clinicians now treat cases with functional appliances which will require extractions as part of their orthodontic therapy. It has been suggested that the extraction pattern may be somewhat different with functional appliance therapy as opposed to removable or fixed therapy of the traditional type. This is for two reasons:

1 Less space is required to achieve overjet reduction since the anterior−posterior discrepancy will have been significantly reduced by the action of the functional appliance.

2 Because the overjet will have been partially reduced during the first phase of treatment less space is required in the lower arch if Class II traction is to be used to complete overjet reduction.

For these reasons the first premolars are less commonly extracted. Second premolars or second molars are often the teeth of choice for extraction.

Treatment of Class II division 1 malocclusion

At the time of initial treatment planning in the young patient who is in the mixed or early permanent dentition, two groups can be identified (Table 7.1):

1 In the first group there is crowding in the lower arch with or without crowding in the upper. In all probability first premolars can be extracted when they have erupted either before or during functional appliance therapy. Suitable appliance modifications must be made to allow for any necessary associated tooth movements to take place within the arches whilst the functional appliance is acting to alter the inter-arch relationship. For example this can be uprighting or distal movement of canines into extraction spaces. In this group of cases only a small proportion can be expected to achieve a satisfactory result without finishing with fixed appliances.

2 In the second group of cases, neither arch demonstrates crowding and in this instance the functional appliance should be fitted and the case regarded initially as a non-extraction one. It is, however, necessary to review the situation in the light of progress.

Table 7.1 Treatment planning of Class II division 1 malocclusion

Skeletal discrepancy	Crowded	Uncrowded
Mild 2	Fixed appliances and extractions	Functional appliance
Moderate 2	Conventional fixed appliance with option of functional to reduce severity	Functional appliance to correct Class II and then review need for extractions—especially at the back of the arch
Severe 2	Premolar extractions with functional appliances followed by fixed appliances, possibly with headgear	Functional appliance and review the need for extractions. Completion with fixed appliance and headgear

One can identify either of two possibilities:

(a) Complete correction of overjet and overbite and a Class I buccal occlusion has been achieved. In these circumstances it may well be wise to consider the need for extraction from the distal end of the arch at the completion of treatment, more as a prophylactic than a therapeutic measure. The choice of extractions will fall from within the second and third molar series of teeth and to some extent this is a controversial issue. Factors which might govern such choice would include the availability of a good oral surgery service as well as the orthodontist's preference. A number of combinations have been suggested such as the removal of all third molars surgically; the removal of all four second molars as a simple extraction procedure; finally the extraction of upper second and lower third molars to eliminate the doubt that surrounds the behaviour of lower third molars after the adjacent second molars have been extracted (Dacre 1987).

(b) In cases where the Class II correction is only partially complete, upper and lower fixed appliances would undoubtedly be required to continue treatment. In this situation it would probably be necessary to extract in the upper arch to gain the necessary space; this would in turn dictate lower arch extractions to balance the occlusion and possibly to provide anchorage. In these circumstances the choice will fall within the premolar group of teeth and the combination of first and/or second premolars extractions may be dictated by the operator's preference or the particular anchorage requirements at this stage of treatment. Frequently the second premolars will be the extraction of choice.

FIRST MOLAR EXTRACTIONS

At a time when enforced extraction of first molars was common it was found that functional appliances were particularly appropriate for the correction of a Class II division 1 incisor relationship after such extractions. This is because treatment can be commenced before the eruption of other permanent teeth, particularly the second molars. By contrast any other conventional procedure usually has to be delayed until these teeth are available for anchorage. Thus the functional appliance option should still be borne in mind when first molar prognosis is in doubt in Class II cases (Fig. 7.4).

The treatment of Class II division 2 malocclusions

Only a small proportion of Class II division 2 malocclusion are appropriate to the treatment by functional appliance therapy alone. It would be necessary for the lower arch to demonstrate virtually perfect or at least acceptable alignment at the commencement of treatment and the crowding and local irregularity in the upper anterior region should not be marked. Since few malocclusions fall into such a convenient group it must be anticipated that virtually all will require treatment at some stage with fixed appliances (Fig. 7.5). For this reason many operators feel that functional appliance therapy has a role in the relatively early mixed dentition phase. Such early treatment can be useful in reducing the incisor overbite and achieving as much Class II correction as possible while awaiting prior to the eruption of the remaining permanent teeth and fixed appliance therapy. This is particularly appropriate when there is evidence of gingival trauma.

Treatment of Class III malocclusion

The treatment of Class III malocclusions with functional appliances is still a controversial issue. There is no doubt that useful dentoalveolar tilting of the upper and lower labial segments can be achieved with a variety of functional appliances and it might be appropriate to attempt this during the mixed dentition phase in order to establish a normal incisor relationship, if this seems attainable. This might obviate the need for an early phase of fixed appliance therapy to be followed by a longish intermediate period of retention before definitive treatment can be instituted with the eruption of the permanent teeth.

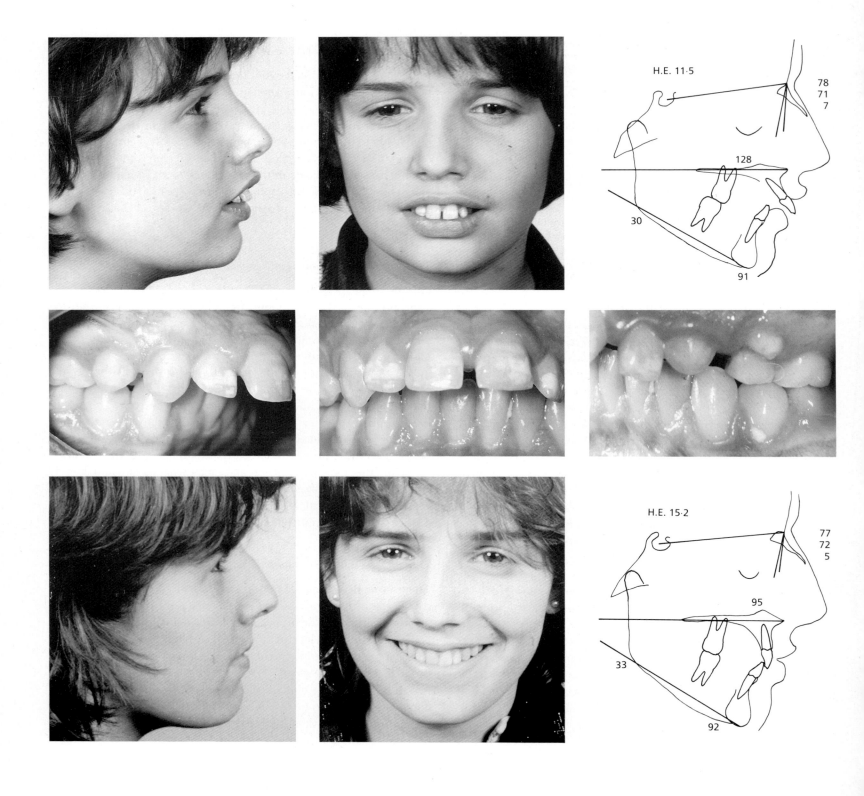

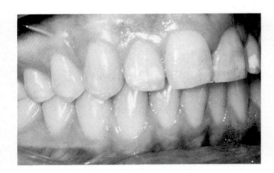 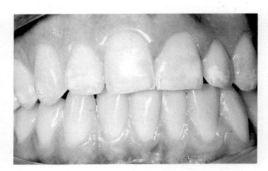 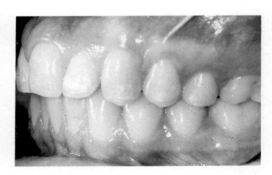

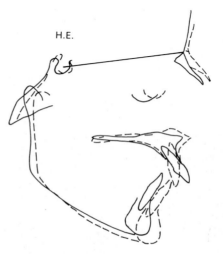

Fig. 7.3 H.E.: A Class II division 1 malocclusion with an overjet of 14 mm treated with an activator–headgear combination and the extraction of upper second and lower third molars.

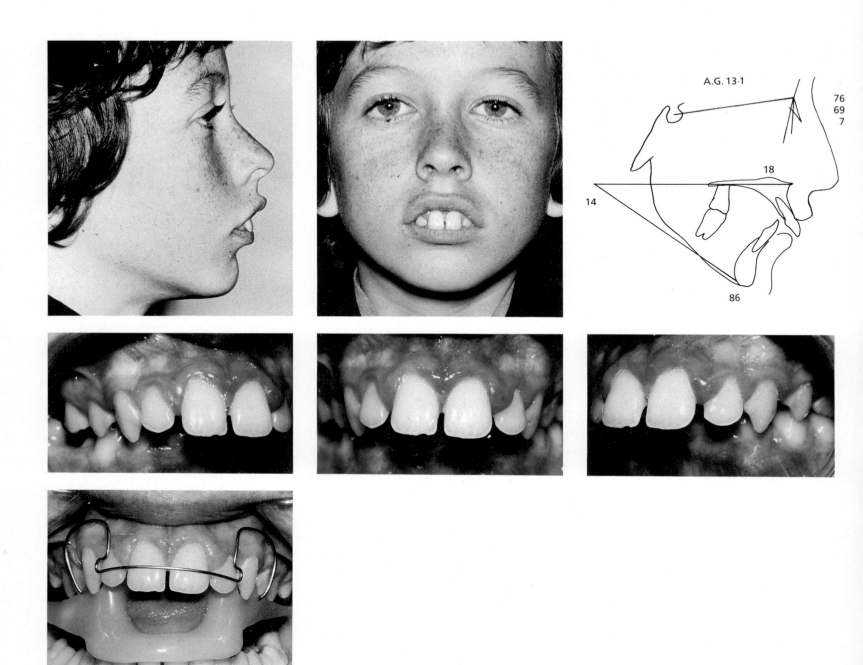

Fig. 7.4 A.G.: A high-angle case. Four first permanent molars were extracted and the malocclusion was treated with an activator alone.

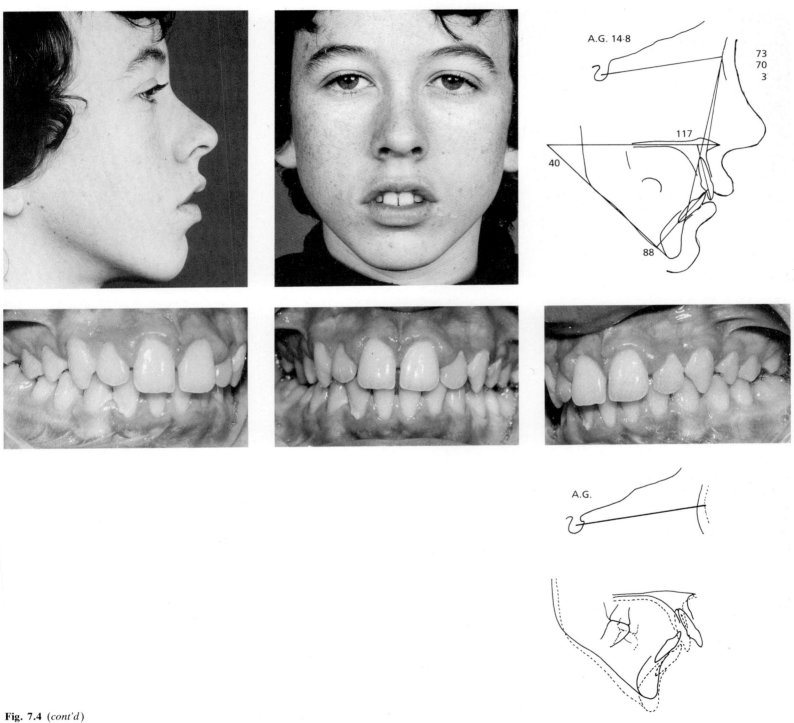

Fig. 7.4 (*cont'd*)

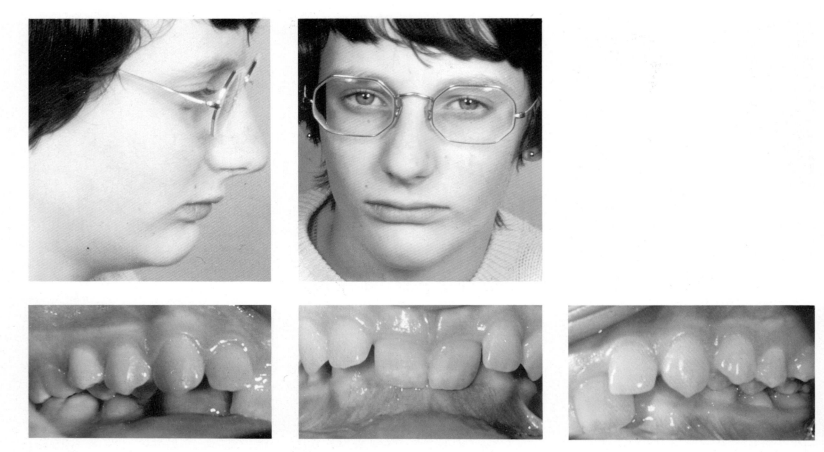

Fig. 7.5 D.S.: A severe Class II division 2 malocclusion with buccal occlusion of the upper premolars. The lower right first premolar had been extracted before the patient presented for treatment. An upper removable appliance was used to reduce the overbite and procline the central incisors. This was followed by an activator to correct the inter-arch relationship. Final alignment was with fixed appliances. The records are shown 3 years out of retention.

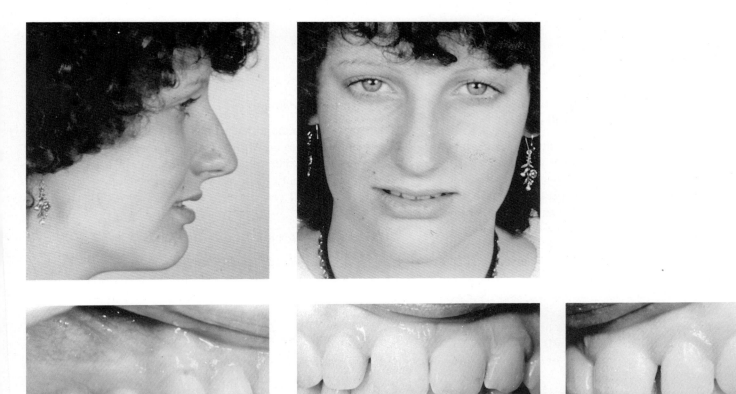

Fig. 7.5 (*cont'd*)

References

Broadbent, J.M. (1987) Correspondence in *American Journal of Orthodontics*, **92**, 75.

Dacre, J.T. (1987) The criteria for lower second molar extraction. *British Journal of Orthodontics*, **1**, 1.

Teuscher, U. (1978) A growth-related concept for Skeletal Class 2 treatment. *American Journal of Orthodontics*, **74**, 258.

Further reading

Levin, K.I. (1985) Activator headgear therapy. *American Journal of Orthodontics*, **87**, 91.

Van Beek, H. (1982) Combined headgear and activator treatment. *European Journal of Orthodontics*, **4**, 279.

Chapter 8   Problems of Research

Problems surrounding investigations into the effectiveness and mode of action of functional appliances

Despite an extensive literature there is still little agreement about the mode of action of functional appliances. This is because, as in any rapidly developing field, there are a large number of conflicting studies and a wide variation in the interpretation which experts place upon them. It is important that the reader has some idea of the difficulties and pitfalls surrounding research into functional appliance treatment, both to understand the reason for the present confusion and in order that he or she may be better equipped to evaluate new research as this becomes available.

The clinical effects of a functional appliance could be ascribed to one or more of the following:
1 Dento-alveolar changes in one or both arches.
2 A restriction or redirection of the growth of the maxilla.
3 A change in the amount or direction of mandibular growth.
4 Remodelling of the glenoid fossa.

It is very difficult to draw up a consensus view of how important each effect is thought to be. This is simply because no such consensus exists. Nevertheless the authors would suggest that the following is the present position.

1 Dento-alveolar changes

It is generally agreed that these form a major part of the treatment effect.

2 Restriction/redirection of maxillary growth

It is accepted that forward growth of the maxilla can be changed by the appliance in a similar manner to that achieved by headgear. Most studies have used alveolar points from which to define changes in the position of the maxilla. To what extent these favourable changes remain in the long term, and whether they are 'skeletal' or 'alveolar', is less widely agreed.

3 Changes in the amount and direction of mandibular growth

Whilst increases in mandibular length of the order of a millimetre have been shown to occur during the treatment of Class II cases, many dispute whether these are any more than transient effects on the inherited pattern of growth. No reduction of mandibular growth in Class III cases is believed to occur.

4 Changes in the form of the glenoid fossa

Beneficial therapeutic changes have been shown to occur in some animal experiments. Recently the first human studies have appeared to support this view.

Research methods

Research into the mode of action of functional appliances falls into two categories, animal studies and human studies, each with its own advantages and disadvantages both to the research worker and the clinician.

Animal studies

Until recently, animal studies have been subject to less stringent ethical restrictions than research on human subjects. It has been relatively easy to obtain fairly large numbers of genetically similar animals which can be kept under carefully controlled conditions. It is therefore possible to be more certain that differences observed between experimental and control animals are the result of the effects of appliances rather than differences between the animals themselves.

This is not to say that such research is easy either in its execution or interpretation. Anaesthetic deaths are quite common in small animals and these may upset carefully selected groups unless allowance is made for this eventuality. Also the effect of operative procedure on the growth of the experimental animal must be taken into consideration. Usually this is achieved by subjecting all the control animals to the same operative procedure as those in the experimental group apart from one clearly defined step which forms the subject of the study. Even so, where surgery is carried out great care must be exercised to ensure that differences between control and experimental groups are due to the procedure being studied and not the result of some associated effect such as surgical scarring or the loss of integrity of adjacent structures (nerves, muscles, etc.).

Whilst the results of carefully controlled animal experiments may have relevance to clinical practice they must always be interpreted with great caution. There are considerable differences between the anatomy of the cranial base, upper face and mandible of man and other mammals. These differences are important because it is agreed that functional appliances achieve their greatest effects in the growing patient and are therefore partly dependent on the pattern of facial growth. To some extent these facial differences can be overcome by using monkeys as the animal model although numbers are almost invariably small because of the much greater cost. Even amongst the primates, however, man is unique in having a chin with the lower incisors and their alveolar process growing more or less vertically. Furthermore, in the upper part of the human face the sutures are set more vertically than in other primates.

Even if these limitations are accepted, other problems remain. Firstly the functional appliance, which is loose fitting in the human and generally worn only part-time, must be cemented or wired into place in animal studies. Secondly the sagittal discrepancies which the functional appliance is used to correct are virtually absent in the animal kingdom. It is unreasonable to suppose that the histological and anatomical changes induced by an appliance which causes Class III malrelation to appear in the jaws of an experimental animal are the same as those which correct a Class II discrepancy in the human.

Human studies

All the limitations mentioned above can be overcome if studies are confined to human subjects. Unfortunately, a whole new series of problems then arise. Study methods are very limited; histological methods, for example, cannot be used. Many early papers contained little more than the clinical opinions of their authors. Later studies have relied extensively upon lateral skull radiographs. Nowadays radiography must usually be limited to those films which can be said to be essential for the proper treatment of the patient. Until recently it has not been possible using lateral skull radiography to separate 'dento-alveolar' and 'basal' (or skeletal) changes. This is because these areas of bone are neither morphologically nor radiographically distinct. More recently the use of metallic implants has done much to clarify the relative contribution of changes occurring in different regions of the same bone. However, the use of implants is limited in many countries by ethical considerations and the number of subjects involved in such studies is usually quite small.

Human studies of the effects of functional appliances can be divided into two categories:

1   Those based upon comparison between a control group and a treatment group.

2   Those comparing before and after records of the same patients.

In the first category the only way to obtain suitable controls is to withhold treatment from subjects whose malocclusion justifies treatment. It is unsatisfactory for example to use a control group of untreated cases with ideal developing dentitions: to do so is as unacceptable as attempting to judge the effect of a fertilizer on the growth of carrots by comparing their weight gain with that of a sample of parsnips.

Even when a control group is used which presents the same type of malocclusion, it must be remembered that patterns of human facial growth differ between the sexes. Control cases must therefore be carefully matched by age and sex to correspond to the subjects found in the treatment group. The number of subjects in both groups must be reasonably large, say 30 or more, to minimize the effects of chance inclusion of very rare, atypical individuals. Clearly such control groups are almost impossible to find these days in Westernized societies except amongst those patients who for some reason have declined treatment. Those who do so may well have less severe malocclusions, or may receive treatment by another method. Also, if they have declined treatment of any kind they will usually be unwilling to attend for subsequent examinations and radiography. A variation is to use control groups in which treatment of a different type was carried out. However, since the treatment is directed to the same end, namely correction of the malocclusion, this approach will obscure some treatment effects. Furthermore it may be difficult to decide whether the differences which are identified are due to functional treatment or the treatment changes produced in the group which is acting as a control.

In the second category (comparing pre- and post-treatment changes) a similar problem arises. Are the changes due to the

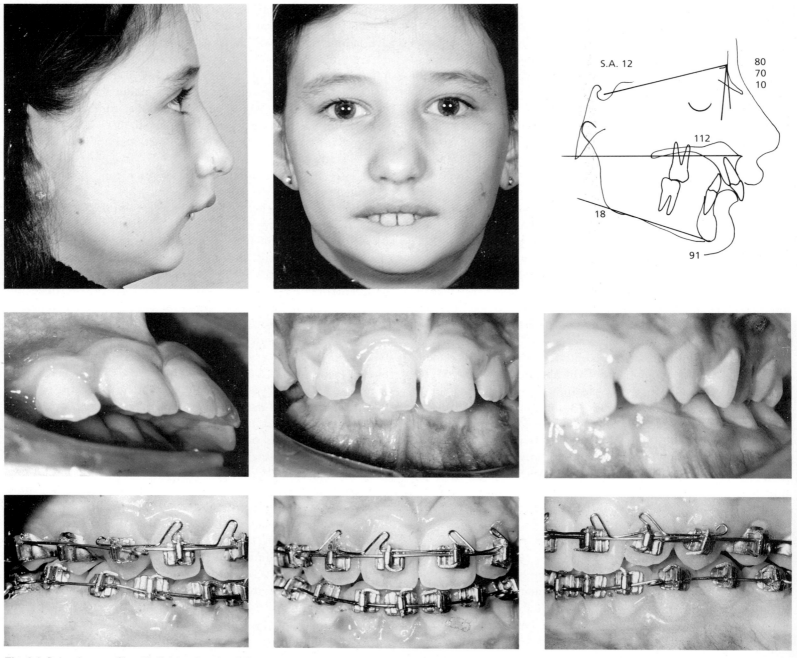

Fig. 8.1 S.A.: A gross Class II division 1 malocclusion with an overjet of 11 mm and an overbite of 12 mm treated with an activator–headgear combination and treatment completed with a fixed appliance on a non-extraction basis. Final records are shown 4 years after the completion of treatment.

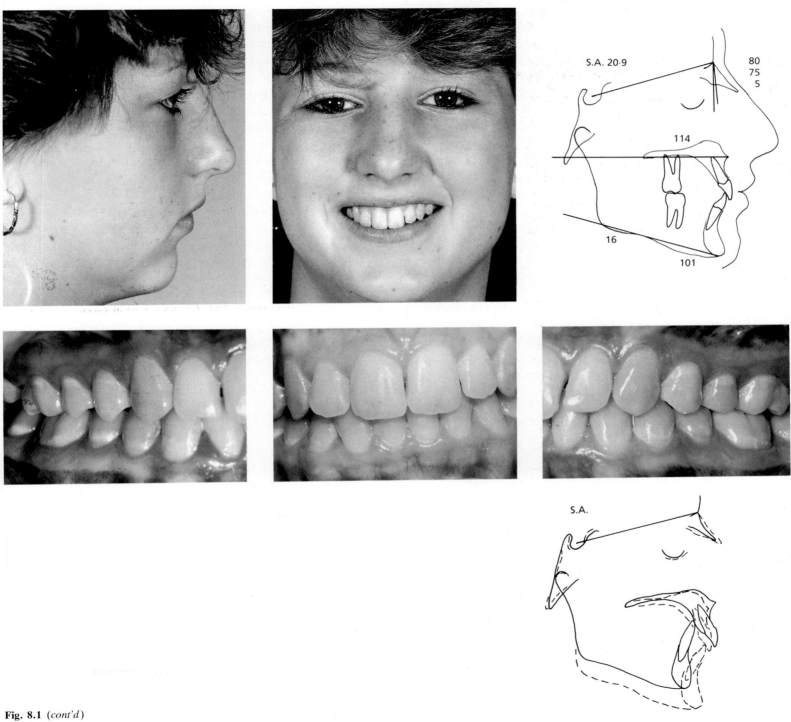

Fig. 8.1 (*cont'd*)

action of the appliance or would they have occurred to some extent anyway? This uncertainty is particularly great where the measurements being compared are derived from the records of successfully treated patients. The impartial observer might reasonably ask whether such a group contains a high proportion of individuals who have shown a particularly favourable (and maybe most unusual) response to treatment. The only way the sceptic can be convinced is when he is presented with large numbers of consecutively treated patients regardless of the outcome of treatment. Whilst the enthusiast may resent such an unbelieving audience, the burden of proof for any new technique rests with those who would wish to see the method more widely adopted.

A further problem, which is particularly noticeable with appliances which use functional principles, is the vast number of small variations in appliance design which are described. Perhaps this may be best illustrated by one aspect of the Andresen appliance. Initially, in the 1930s, there appear to have been no hard and fast rules concerning the production of the construction bite for this appliance. At first small inter-occlusal distances were used which were secondary to the more important consideration of forward displacement of the mandible. Over subsequent years the vertical displacement of the mandible was increased, perhaps due to clinical experience and perhaps to prevent rejection of the appliance during sleep. With these wider opening appliances forward displacement of the lower jaw is severely restricted. In other words, horizontal displacement, in many clinicians' minds, is now secondary to vertical opening. Because the relative importance of these and other minor variations have remained largely uninvestigated it is hardly surprising that conflicting conclusions on the effectiveness of functional appliances abound in the literature.

Even where properly conducted, human studies with carefully selected controls have shown that functional appliances can produce beneficial changes which are statistically significant (i.e. it has been established beyond reasonable doubt that these are due to treatment and not due to chance) these changes have usually been very small. Once again our sceptic will ask how much benefit does the millimetre of induced growth in the mandible confer on a Class II case if the discrepancy between the arches is ten times this amount? In other words are such benefits *clinically* significant? The enthusiast will then reply that any improvement is welcome in such cases and that the collective effect of many such small changes in the growing face can add up to a very significant clinical effect (Fig. 8.1).

Appendices

Appendix 1   Summary of Published Papers

This following review of papers covering research into functional appliances is by no means exhaustive. It has been selected mainly from publications written in English and serves to illustrate the range of research to date and often demonstrates conflicting results. A deeper examination of some of the possible reasons for the differing conclusions is outside the scope of this book.

Adenwalla, S.T. & Kronman, J.H. (1985) Class II division 1 treatment with Frankel and Edgewise appliances. *Angle Orthodontist*, **55**, 281–298.

Treatment changes of 20 patients treated with the Frankel appliance (FR2) were compared cephalometrically with 20 treated with 0.018 inch Edgewise mechanics.
Findings: Both groups showed similar improvements with no statistically significant differences in mandibular growth. The increase seen in lower face height during treatment was greater in the Edgewise group although this difference was not statistically significant.

Ahlgren, J. & Laurin, C. (1976) Late results of activator treatment: a cephalometric study. *British Journal of Orthodontics*, **3**, 181–187.

A study of 50 consecutively treated cases of Class II and Class III malocclusions with Andresen appliances constructed according to Andresen & Haupl (1945). The successful and unsuccessful cases were compared.
Findings: Results showed that in successful cases:
1 There was a dental-alveolar change in both upper and lower arches. There was maxillary retardation in Class II and maxillary stimulation in Class III.
2 The mandible was unaffected and there was no tendency to induce posterior rotation of the mandible.
3 There was an increase in lower face height.
4 There was greater ANB discrepancy at the start of treatment than in the unsuccessful cases.
The authors conclude that successful treatment requires good co-operation, high growth intensity, favourable growth pattern and a well-constructed appliance.

Auf der Maur, H.J. (1980) Electro-myographic recordings of the lateral pterygoid muscle in activator treatment of Class II division 1 malocclusion cases. *European Journal of Orthodontics*, **2**, 161–171.

This study was undertaken to clarify the effect of the Herren activator on the mandible and the suprahyoid and lateral pterygoid muscles. Records were obtained from eight patients including a set of monozygotic twins. Implanted electrodes were used for electromyography of these muscles. Difficulty was experienced in locating the electrodes. (Some patients required sedatives and the needle had to be withdrawn temporarily for patients to complete their jaw movements.)
Findings: The author questions the role of lateral pterygoid muscle suggested by other authors (notably Petrovic & McNamara) and agrees with Herren that the activator acts as a passive appliance inducing elastic and myotatic tension in the muscles.

Awn, M., Goret-Nicaise, M. & Dhem. A. (1987) Unilateral section of the lateral pterygoid muscle in the growing rat does not alter condylar growth. *European Journal of Orthodontics*, **9**, 122–128.

This study, involving 360 Sprague Dawley rats, was undertaken to test whether the reduction of mitotic activity in prechodroblasts, observed by Petrovic & Stutzman (1972) following sectioning of the lateral pterygoid, was associated with a reduction in condylar growth. The work involved rats of both sexes from 4 to 6 weeks of age and complements earlier work with 10-week-old animals (Gore-Nicaise *et al.* 1983). Using a tetracyline and alizarin dye marker no significant differences were found between control and experimental groups in the growth of the condylar cartilage.

Baume, L.J. & Derichsweiler, H. (1961) Is the condylar growth centre responsive to orthodontic treatment? *Oral Surgery, Oral Medicine and Oral Pathology*, **14**, 347–362.

Three young monkeys aged 44–50 months were used: one of them as a control, two with upper and lower metal splints to give a habitual forward bite. All were injected with alizarin red S and had sagittal films before and after the experimental period. Monkey 2 was killed at 2 months and Monkey 3 at 4 months. Cephalometric assessment and gross and microscopic examination of the mandible gave the following results.

Findings: Both experimental monkeys showed obvious changes in the gross anatomy and X-ray outline of the head of the condyles which were greatest in the animal killed after 4 months. Histology showed increased cartilage proliferation and endocondyle ossification in a posterior direction.

Baumrind, S., Korn, E.L., Isaacson, R.J., West, E.E. & Molthen, R. (1983) Superimpositional assessment of treatment-associated changes in the temporomandibular joint and the mandibular symphysis. *American Journal of Orthodontics*, **84**, 443–465.

The paper reports on a cephalometric appraisal of 238 Class II patients treated in three different ways: 74 subjects received cervical traction, 53 had high-pull headgear to first molars, 61 were treated with Harvold activators and there were 50 controls.
Findings: It is very difficult to summarize briefly this extremely thorough and detailed investigation which examines overall, annual and treatment-induced changes relative to the anterior cranial base. Perhaps the most intriguing finding is that while the modified activator sample produced a significantly increased rate of growth compared with the controls, similar significant effects were found with the cervical traction group. Small but significant differences were found between these two treatment methods. The activator produced greater changes at pogonion

in the forward direction (compared with controls), whilst the cervical group had greater downward displacement.

van Beek, H. (1982) Overjet correction by a combined headgear and activator. *European Journal of Orthodontics*, **4**, 279–290.

The study is of 40 consecutively treated patients (20 boys, 20 girls aged 9–14 years). All were fitted with a Harvold type of activator incorporating high-pull headgear attachments. There were no controls.

Findings: Generally, overjet reduction was rapidly achieved; in a majority this was fully reduced after 9 months of treatment. In addition to the changes usually associated with activator treatment there was usually intrusion of the upper incisors. Surprisingly, despite efforts to avoid it, proclination of the lower incisors occurred.

Birkbebaek, L., Melsen, B. & Terp, S. (1984) A laminagraphic study of the alterations in the temporo-mandibular joint following activator treatment. *European Journal of Orthodontics*, **6**, 257–266.

Twenty-three children aged 9 to 13 years in the mixed dentition had implants inserted as described by Björk (1968) and received activator treatment according to Harvold (1974). After one month, ten of the children had not used the activator and were used as controls. The effects of the activator in the treated group were studied by means of a standardized method of laminagraphy (12- and 44- degree laminagraphs) and conventional profile radiographs taken before and after treatment (10 months interval).

Findings: The authors found on the basis of their results that it was not possible to reject any of the different opinions on the effect of activator treatment. They conclude that the effects of the activator could be considered as being composed of a multiplicity of factors including most importantly intra-maxillary tooth displacement and changes in the direction and amount of condylar growth. They also note that changes in the slope of the occlusal plane due to differential eruption and remodelling of the articular fossa played a part.

Björk, A. (1951) The principle of Andresen method of orthodontic treatment, a discussion based on cephalometric X-ray analysis of treated cases. *American Journal of Orthodontics*, **37**, 437–458.

Treatment in three types of Class II division 1 and Class III cases is described and illustrated. The advantages and disadvantages of activator treatment are listed.

Bolmgren, G.A. & Moshiri, F. (1986) Bionator treatment in Class II division 1. *Angle Orthodontist*, **56**, 255–262.

Twenty cases (12 males, 8 females) treated with the bionator were compared with a similar number treated with 'fixed appliances' and with a control sample drawn from the University of Michigan growth study. In the bionator group initial treatment was followed by conventional fixed appliance treatment. Sadly, full experimental data is not published in this report but the authors conclude that the most notable difference produced by the bionator was an increase in the vertical dimension and mandibular plane angle.

Bookstein, F.L. (1983) Measuring treatment effects on craniofacial growth. In: McNamara, J.A., Ribben, K.A. & Howe, R.P. (eds), *Clinical alteration of the growing face*. Monograph 14, Centre for Human Growth and Development, University of Michigan.

The author believes that conventional methods of quantifying treatment-induced changes are inappropriate to describe changes of form. His method examines the transformation of triangles based on conventional cephalometric landmarks. Large samples are used to examine the effects of the Harvold activator, the Frankel appliance and cervical traction.

Findings: It is difficult to do justice to this thought-provoking paper. Perhaps the most important immediate finding is that conventional measures of mandibular length and lower face height are inappropriate to study the effects of myofunctional appliances as they are not made in the plane of greatest change. The author also reports similar effects on the lower face with all three treatment methods although the horizontal and vertical changes differed in each. Cervical traction also produced a downward and backward rotational effect of the line sella–ANS, which was not seen with the other treatments.

Carels, C. & van der Linden, P.M.G. (1987) Concepts of functional appliances' mode of action. *American Journal of Orthodontics*, **92**, 162–168.

A very thorough review of the evidence supporting the various hypotheses of the modes of action of functional appliances. The authors finally propose their own hypothesis based on their neuromuscular measurements in children treated with the bionator (Carels, C. & van Steenberghe, D. (1986) *American Journal of Orthodontics*, **90**, 410–419). This work does not indicate a need for the gradual advancement of the mandible during myofunctional treatment but rather that the larger the forward displacement the larger the neuromuscular response.

Clark, W.J. (1982) The twin block traction technique. *European Journal of Orthodontics*, **4**, 129–138.

A description by its originator of this technique, illustrated by records of two treated Class II division 1 cases.

Clark, W.J. (1988) Twin block technique. *American Journal of Orthodontics*, **93**, 1–18.

This gives an account of this treatment method, illustrated by the records of four treated Class II division 1 cases, two of which include cephalometric tracings. Although the author summarizes the results of a cephalometric study of 70 consecutively treated twin block cases, no data for these are given.

Creekmore, T.D. & Radney, L.J. (1983) Frankel appliance therapy: orthopedic or orthodontic? *American Journal of Orthodontics* **83**, 89–108.

Purpose of this study was to examine the capability of the Frankel appliance to elicit a differential growth response. All material was successfully treated in one practice.

Findings: Class II cases (11 subjects) showed no more mandibular forward growth than Class I cases (9 subjects). Furthermore, treated cases grew no more than the untreated subjects (62 controls, 50 Edgewise-treated controls). They question the precept that forward posture stimulates mandibular growth in man. Forward growth of the maxilla was significantly reduced in the Class II Frankel sample compared with untreated, but not with Edgewise-treated. Class II correction with Frankel was achieved by 37% orthodontic retraction of the upper incisors; 26% labial movement of the lower incisors; 16% retraction of maxilla and 21% normal mandibular forward growth. Both Frankel and Edgewise appliance change the direction of the condyle to a more upwards and backwards direction (unfavourably) and many skeletal changes attributed to treatment were observed in untreated cases and in Edgewise-treated cases.

DeGroote, C.W. (1984) Alterability of mandibular condylar growth in the young rat and its implications. *Thesis*, Leuven, Belgium.

This work contains a good review of animal experiments on the subject. The author's original work concerns the effect of:
1 intermittent (12 hours per day) and continuous enforced forward displacement;
2 continuous enforced lateral displacement in 28-day-old Wistar rat.
Findings: In the forward displacement groups (30 subjects in each and 30 controls) condylar and mandibular growth has slowed. There was a gradual recovery in the rate of vertical growth, and to a lesser extent horizontal growth, in those animals who had full-time wear of the appliance. Horizontal growth rates did not recover in the intermittent-wear group. In the lateral displacement experiment (10 animals and 10 controls) there was generally increased growth on the side on which there was forward displacement on the condyle whilst on the contralateral side growth was reduced.

Emmerson, W. (1982) Activator growth augmentation — a long term perspective. *Thesis*, Loma Linda University.

Twenty-three activator patients were followed through to age 18. They were evaluated at three intervals: before, after and 5 years following treatment. No other appliances were used for the Class II correction. The findings were compared with the predicted growth provided by the Ricketts Rocky Mountain Data Services (11 factors).
Findings: The results indicated a significant increase in growth in the brachyfacial patients over that expected. Most of the increased growth was vertical at the condyle and in this area. There was no inhibition of maxillary growth, no post-treatment fall-off in the growth spurt and virtually no relapse of the molar relationship.

Eirew, H.L., McDowell, F. & Phillips, J.G. (1982) Frankel appliance therapy — avoidance of lower incisor proclination. *British Journal of Orthodontics*, **8**, 189–190.

The authors claim that this undesirable tooth movement is brought about by incorrect design, construction and use of the Frankel appliance.

Elgoyhen, J.C., Moyers, R.E., McNamara, J.A. & Riolo, M.L. (1972) Craniofacial adaptation to protrusive function in young rhesus monkeys. *American Journal of Orthodontics*, **62**, 469–480.

Sixteen juvenile rhesus monkeys were fitted with appliances to promote forward posturing of the mandible. Three animals had unilateral and three bilateral appliances, ten acted as controls. All animals had tantalum pins implanted in maxilla and mandible. Results were evaluated using serial lateral cephalograms.

Findings:
1 After appliances were removed all experimental animals demonstrated mandibular prognathism and a Class III molar relationship.
2 Statistically significant increases in the rate and amount of growth at the head of the condyle were recorded.
3 There was more forward and less vertical growth of the maxilla in the experimental group.
4 Dento-alveolar changes were also observed.

Enlow, D.H., Digangi, D., MacNamara, J.A. Jr & Mina, M. (1988) An evaluation of the morphogenic and anatomic effects of the functional (sic) regulator utilizing the counterpart analysis. *European Journal of Orthodontics*, **10**, 192–202.

This is a report of the effects of the function regulator in the treatment of 96 subjects (mean age 10 years 2 months) compared with 41 untreated controls. The analysis compares regional anatomical relationships cephalometrically using a 'goodness of fit' technique. The authors describe differences in response which they believe could lead to better prediction of results of treatment through the identification of different Class II craniofacial types.

Forsberg, C.M. & Odenrick, L. (1981) Skeletal and soft tissue response to activator treatment. *European Journal of Orthodontics*, **3**, 247–253.

Forty-seven Andresen cases successfully treated were compared with 31 untreated Class II division 1 controls matched for age, sex and facial morphology.
Findings: The reduction in ANB angle in the treated group (1.4 degrees) was significantly greater than in the untreated group (0.3 degrees) ($P < 0.01$). SNA decreased during treatment but increased in the untreated group. There was no significant difference in SNB increase between the two groups. The overjet reduced in the treated group and was unchanged in the untreated group ($P < 0.001$). The occlusal results were satisfactory but profile changes were not improved in all instances.

Frankel, R. (1970) Maxillary retrusion in Class III and treatment with the Function Corrector III. *Transactions of the European Orthodontic Society*, **46**, 249–259.

A description of the principles of the FR3 is followed by a comparative study of Class III cases treated by FR1 and FR3 appliances.
Findings: The author concludes that the FR3 appliance produces significant maxillary forward growth when the results are compared with (a) untreated Class II cases and (b) Class II cases treated with FR1 appliances. However, both the control groups and the reference point chosen are rather unusual and the results are therefore difficult to interpret.

Frankel, R. (1971) The guidance of eruption without extraction. *Transactions of the European Orthodontic Society*, **47**, 303–316.

This is an early account of the effect of the function regulator upon dental development. Two illustrative cases are included.

Frankel, R. & Frankel, C. (1983) A functional approach to the treatment of open bite. *American Journal of Orthodontics*, **84**, 54–68.

This is an account of possible use of the function regulator in the treatment of openbite. A sample of 30 treated cases were compared with 11 controls whose openbites had remained untreated. Measurements were obtained on serial cephalometric radiographs taken over a period of 8 years, analysed by means of the method of Nahoum, Jarabak and Frankel.
Findings: With the Frankel analysis significant differences in vertical skeletal development were found between treated and non-treated groups. The authors conclude that the striking improvement in facial appearance may result as much from changes in the soft tissue mask as from skeletal changes.

Freunthaller, P. (1967) Cephalometric observations in Class II division 1 malocclusions treated with the activator. *Angle Orthodontist*, **37**, 18–25.

Thirty-five successfully treated patients with the activator. The cephalometric assessment was based on the maxillary plane. A line was drawn from this plane through A-point to the pogonion, and the angle thus formed designated MM.
Findings: This angle showed a significant increase during treatment due to the pogonion coming forwards which showed a correlation with increase in length of the body of the mandible. There was no control in this series but a comparison was made with the published work of Frolich which showed that there was no sagittal improvement in untreated Class II cases although this study was done entirely on models.

Ghafari, J. & Heeley, J.D. (1982) Condylar adaption to muscle alteration in the rat. *Angle Orthodontist*, **52**, 26–37.

The effect of detaching the right masseter muscle was studied histologically in 25- and 60-day-old Holtzman rats. In one group the muscle was left to re-attach spontaneously and in another it was repositioned as far anteriorly as possible.
Findings: The results indicated that the alteration in muscle function led to a rapid change in the morphology of both condyles. Histological appearances suggested that homeostasis was achieved in about 50 days.

Gianelly, A.A., Arena, S.A. & Bernstein, I. (1984) A comparison of Class II treatment changes noted with the light wire, edgewise and Frankel appliances. *American Journal of Orthodontics*, **86**, 269–276.

Cephalometric records of three groups of patients were compared. Each subgroup comprised ten males and six or seven females whose Class II malocclusions had been treated with either Edgewise, Begg or Frankel appliances.
Findings: Despite the fact that the Frankel group represented the 16 most successfully treated cases the annual rate of increase of the mandibular length

(Ar–Gn) was similar in all three groups and there were no statistically significant differences found between the changes obtained by the three treatment techniques.

Graber, T.M., Rakosi, T. & Petrovic, A. (1985) *Dentofacial Orthopaedics with Functional Appliances*, 449. C.V. Mosby, St Louis.

This volume is the result of collaboration between three well known and prolific writers from two continents. They have produced a comprehensive text on myofunctional appliances, aimed principally at the American orthodontist and postgraduate student. This is a very valuable book, not the least for its excellent list of references for further reading. Its only weakness is its rather sketchy coverage of the results of clinical research.

Hagg, U. & Pancherz, H. (1988) Dentofacial orthopaedics in relation to chronological age, growth period and skeletal development. An analysis of 72 male patients treated with the Herbst appliance. *European Journal of Orthodontics*, **10**, 169–176.

This retrospective cephalometric study concludes:
1 That skeletal contribution to Class II correction during orthopaedic treatment will be greatest in patients treated around peak height velocity.
2 Chronological age cannot be used to estimate mandibular growth capacity; velocity growth curves of standing height are the most useful aid for doing this.
3 Skeletal maturity indicators employing the third phalanx of the middle finder (MP3) also seem to be a useful aid for estimating mandibular growth capacity.

Hamano, Y. & Ahlgren, J. (1987) A cephalometric study of the construction bite of the activator. *European Journal of Orthodontics*, **9**, 305–313.

In this cephalometric study, 30 children (mean age 10 years 3 months) were divided into two groups determined by pretreatment differences in the construction bite. Within each group the cases were consecutively treated. In group 1 separation of the incisors was from 1 to 3 mm, whilst in group 2 the incisors were held edge to edge. The authors conclude that a significantly larger sagittal displacement of the mandible occurred in group 2 cases. The effects of this upon treatment will be reported in due course.

Harvold, E.P. & Vargevic, K. (1971) Morphogenetic response to activator treatment. *American Journal of Orthodontics*, **60**, 478–490.

Twenty treatment subjects treated with the Harvold activator and 20 controls (not matched for age or sex) were compared. The treatment group was significantly older than the controls but there were no significant skeletal differences.
Findings: The study was carried out to test the following hypotheses:
1 Is there an increase in the growth of the mandible? Answer: no.
2 Is there forward migration of the mandibular teeth? Answer: no.
3 Is there reduced forward growth of the maxilla? Answer: probably.
4 Is there distal migration of the maxillary teeth? Answer: no.
5 Is there an increase in the height of the mandibular alveolus? Answer: probably.
   In addition it was found that there was increased growth in face height and lingual tipping of the upper incisors.

Haynes, S. (1986) A cephalometric study of mandibular changes in modified function regulator (Frankel) treatment. *American Journal of Orthodontics*, **90**, 308–320.

A group of 29 (16 boys, 13 girls) Class II division 1 cases treated with a modified function regulator (FR1) was compared with a similar number of matched controls. A comparison of pre- and post-treatment radiographs demonstrated highly significant differences in the following mandibular dimensions: (1) articulare/B point; (2) articulare/mandibular incisal edge; (3) gonion/B-point; (4) gonion/mandibular incisal edge; (5) occlusal plane length; (6) posterior border/mandibular incisal edge. The mean differences were between 2 and 3 mm greater in the treated group than in the control group.

Haynes, S. (1986) Profile changes in modified function regulator therapy. *Angle Orthodontist*, **56**, 309–314.

An experimental group of 31 Class II division 1 patients (15 male, 13 female, mean age 109.8 months, mean treatment duration 41 months) were compared with an untreated control group of 28 subjects (9 male, 19 female, mean age 104.3 months, mean observation time 37.9 months). Cephalometric comparisons were made with respect to the anterior nasal plane (a tangent drawn through the tip of the nose running perpendicular to the ANS/PNS plane).

The author concludes that there are clinically significant antero-posterior changes associated with function regulator treatment but that these are limited to the incisor teeth of both arches and their associated soft tissues. No statistically significant differences were found between mandibular skeletal landmarks and the anterior nasal plane.

Heij, D.G.O., Callaert, H. & Opdebeeck, H.M. (1989) The effect of the amount of protrusion built in to the Bionator on condylar growth and displacement: a clinical study. *American Journal of Orthodontics*, **95**, 401–409.

This is a cephalometric study of 14 Class II division 1 patients (6 male, 8 female, mean age 10 years 3 months) treated for one year with bionators. One group had an edge to edge bite maintained throughout treatment, the other had a maxi-propulsion bite (after Chateau 1955).

Findings:
1 The nature and magnitude of the treatment effects of the two approaches differ significantly.
2 Increasing the amount of protrusion beyond the edge to edge position did not result in increased ramal growth but appeared to be more effective in treating the sagittal relationship, possibly through a more downward and forward displacement of the condyle.
3 The effect on the condyle positioning appeared to occur mainly in boys.
4 The orthopaedic effect in the maxilla was greater in the edge to edge group.
They suggest that in future studies of this kind boys and girls should be considered separately.

Hinton, J. & McNamara, J.A. Jr (1984) Temporal bone adaptations in response to protrusive function in juvenile and young adult rhesus monkeys. *European Journal of Orthodontics*, **6**, 155–174.

Temporal bone adaptations to protrusive function were studied in 28 juvenile and 19 young adult monkeys (*Macaca mulatta*).

Findings: In the juveniles, adaptive changes were seen in the joint. The most pronounced involved new bone being deposited in the posterior region of the fossa. Response in adults was slower and much more variable but qualitatively similar changes to that of juveniles were seen in one-third of the sample.

Janson, I. (1977) A cephalometric study of the efficiency of the bionator. *Transactions of the European Orthodontic Society*, **53**, 283–293.

A study of 207 subjects with Class II malocclusion (134 treated with bionator and 73 controls). Comparisons were made for eight subgroups, divided according to skeletal maturity and facial form.

Findings:
1 The bionator had no significant effect on natural growth pattern of the face.
2 There were significant dento-alveolar effects, for example the inter-incisal angle was significantly increased in the treatment group. Greater effects were noted in the pubertal period.
3 The horizontal discrepancies were reduced to a greater extent by retrusion of the upper incisors than by protrusion of the lowers.

Kantomaa, T. (1984) Effect of increased upward displacement of the glenoid fossa on mandibular growth. *European Journal of Orthodontics*, **6**, 183–191.

Vertical growth of the mandibular condyle was studied in 28 rabbits by inducing an artificially increased upward displacement of the glenoid fossa.

Findings: The results suggested that the adaptability of the condylar cartilage in the rabbit expresses itself mainly in a change in the direction of growth. The work does not support the hypothesis that vertical growth of the mandible is the result of downward pull of the mandible.

Kantomaa, T. & Ronning, O. (1982) The effect of electrical stimulation of the lateral pterygoid muscle on the growth of mandible in the rat. *Proceedings of the Finnish Dental Society*, **78**, 215–219.

Twenty-eight 30-day-old rats were used as experimental animals.

Findings: After 16 days the left side of the mandible was significantly longer than that on the right. These measurements were taken from the condyle to either the mental foramen or the symphysis. There was no increase in the vertical dimension.

Knight, H. (1988) The effects of three methods of orthodontic appliance therapy on some commonly used cephalometric variables. *American Journal of Orthodontics*, **93**, 237–244.

Ninety Class II division 1 cases (30 Begg, 30 Andresen, and 30 Headgear) were compared with each other and with 17 untreated controls using cephalometric radiographs taken pre and post treatment and at least 12 months post retention.

Findings:
1 Andresens did not produce significant change in angle SNA although Begg and Headgear treatment did.
2 Andresen and Headgear treatment did not produce any greater change in SN/MxP than was seen in the controls.
3 Begg and Headgear treatment indirectly prevented the increase in angle SNB seen in the untreated controls. This was through causing a rotation of the mandible with an increase in the angle SN/MdP. The Andresen did not produce this effect.
4 Although the Begg and Headgear therapy produced a downward and backward rotation of the mandible which was reflected in the angle SN/MdP, this was transitory and none of the treatment methods permanently affected this variable.

Korkhaus, G. (1960) Present orthodontic thought in Germany: experiences with the Norwegian method of functional orthopedics in the treatment of distocclusion. *American Journal of Orthodontics*, **46**, 270–274.

An early discussion on the activator and its advantages, disadvantages and uses with some illustrated cases.

Lehman, R., Romuli, A., Bakker, V. (1988) Five year treatment results with a headgear-activator combination. *European Journal of Orthodontics*, **10**, 309–318.

This is a study of the treatment and five-year follow-up changes of a group of 23 Class II division 1 cases treated with the headgear activator combination described by Lehman (1984). Relapse occurred in four patients and was related to posterior growth rotation (as revealed by the y-axis) both during and after treatment. There was no change in the direction of growth rotation seen during treatment and during the follow-up period.

Luder, H.U. (1981) The effects of activator treatment—evidence for the occurrence of two different types of reaction. *European Journal of Orthodontics*, **3**, 205–222.

This study is of 12 male and 13 female patients with matching controls, all aged about 9 years at the start of treatment. The experimental group were Class II division 1 (the nature of the control was not disclosed).
Findings: There was a significant difference in the growth increments of control male and females and therefore the sexes were analysed separately.
1 (*Males*) The amount and direction of condylar growth are altered by the appliance, the displacement of the maxilla is not influenced but there is pronounced inhibition of vertical dental development so that the bony chin grows forwards to an increased extent but the direction of growth is unchanged.
2 (*Females*) Condylar growth is redirected more posteriorly but downward and forward growth of the maxilla is inhibited. Inhibition vertically is less marked and so the mandible is rotated downwards and backwards.
The findings could be explained either by a different reaction or growth pattern in boys and girls or by differences in the height of construction bites used.

Luder, H.U. (1982). Skeletal and profile changes related to two patterns of activator effects. *American Journal of Orthodontics*, **81**, 390–396.

Findings: In the re-analysis of earlier results the author argues that the different responses seen in boys and girls are due to differences in height of the construction bites. (The higher construction bite was used unintentionally in males because of their deeper initial overbite.)

Macdonald, F. (1987) The effect of articular function on the mandibular condyle of the rat. *European Journal of Orthodontics*, **9**, 87–96.

This is a report of an autoradiographic and histological study of 57 Wistar albino rats. There were two experimental procedures. In one the zygomatic arch was removed; in the other the zygomatic arch and articular disc were removed. In each group a sham operation was performed on the animal's contralateral side in which the zygomatic arch was merely exposed.
The author concludes that:
1 Articular function is important in maintaining the organization of the condylar cartilage.
2 The disc and capsule are important constraints on the condylar head and maintain condylar form.
3 There is no evidence that loss of articular function impedes condylar growth.

McDougall, P.D., McNamara, J.A. Jr & Dierkes, J.M. (1982) Arch width development in Class II patients treated with Frankel appliances. *American Journal of Orthodontics*, **82**, 10–22.

Sixty Class II division 1 patients treated by means of Frankel FR1 and FR2 appliances were compared with 47 untreated Class II division 1 controls. Short-term (12–30 months) and long-term (31–48 months) changes were compared using callipers to measure dental casts.

Findings:
1 Expansion of upper and lower dental arches and their supporting structures occurs routinely with the FR1 and FR2 when the appliance is worn conscientiously.
2 The expansion is not limited to a particular region.
3 In the maxilla narrow arches tend to expand more than wider arches.
Stability of these changes is not covered.
Note: The control group showed an increase in molar width during the observation period. Owen's control group from RMDS included no such change (see below).

McNamara, J.A. Jr (1984) Dentofacial adaptions in adult patients following functional regulator therapy. *American Journal of Orthodontics*, **85**, 57–71.

A report of the treatment of three cases by means of the function regulator of Frankel (FR2). Despite patient co-operation being excellent only minimal skeletal and dental changes were observed and in each case these were insufficient to completely resolve the malocclusion.

McNamara, J.A. Jr, Bookstein, F.L. & Shaughnessy, T.G. (1985) Skeletal and dental changes following functional regulator therapy on Class II patients. *American Journal of Orthodontics*, **88**, 91–110.

Records of 100 patients, treated by eight clinicians using Frankel FR2 appliances, were compared with the records of 41 untreated Class II cases. Both conventional and 'tensor analysis' (Bookstein 1983) was used.

Findings:
1 The appliance had little effect on the maxillary skeletal structures.
2 The forward but not the vertical growth of the first molar was reduced.
3 There was some lingual tipping of the upper incisors and some forward tipping of the lowers.
4 There was increased vertical eruption of the lower molars and substantial advancement of these teeth with respect to maxillary structures but not with respect to the mandibular body.
5 There was a marked increase in the lower facial height but not of the facial axis angle or mandibular plane angle.
Note: Using the criteria described for case selection in the method it is likely that a high proportion of successful cases was included in the experimental group.

Madone, G. & Ingervall, B. (1984) Stability of results and function of the masticatory system in patients treated with the Herren type of activator. *European Journal of Orthodontics*, **6**, 92–110.

Forty-nine patients who had been treated with the Herren type of activator were examined between 3 and 8 years out of retention.
Findings: As few patients had pre-treatment cephalograms most conclusions are based on occlusal changes.
1 Reduction of the overjet remained essentially stable after treatment.
2 In half the subjects the overbite increased and in the remainder it decreased somewhat after treatment.
3 In most subjects partial relapse in molar correction occurred out of retention.
4 Prevalence of the symptoms and signs of mandibular dysfunctions were no greater than reported in studies of untreated individuals.

Male, L.R.O. & Tonge, E.A. (1986) A long term follow up of four cases treated with the Andresen appliance. *British Journal of Orthodontics*, **13**, 195–208.

A report of four patients, treated with Andresen appliances, who were recalled 20 years after completion of treatment. It was found that in all cases changes had occurred since the patients were discharged at between 2 and 4 years post-treatment. All cases showed occlusal changes and an increase in facial height.

Marschner, J.F. & Harris, J.E. (1966) The mandibular growth and Class II treatment. *Angle Orthodontist*, **36**, 89–93.

Twelve male Class II division 1 patients (age unspecified) treated with an Andresen/Haupl activator appliance were compared with a control group consisting of 23 untreated Class II patients, age range 5–13 years. The length of the mandible on lateral skull from condyle to symphysis was measured and compared with the control. To overcome the varying intervals of X-rays forwards and backwards extrapolation was used to give monthly increments.

Findings: A statistically significant difference in growth increments between treated and untreated cases was found.

Meach, C.L. (1966) A cephalometric comparison of bony profile changes in Class II division 1 patients treated with extraoral force and functional jaw orthopedics. *American Journal of Orthodontics*, **52**, 353–370.

Thirty Class II division 1 cases treated with a monobloc were compared with an untreated Class I control group and second group consisting of 46 Class II division 1 cases treated with headgear.
Findings: The pogonion came forward more in the monobloc cases than in the headgear and control groups. There was also a closing of the FMPA angle but an increase in the facial angle.

Meikle, M.C. (1970) The effect of a Class II intermaxillary force on the dentofacial complex in the adult *macaca mulatta* monkey. *American Journal of Orthodontics*, **58**, 323–340.

Three adult *Macaca mulatta* monkeys were fitted with Class II intermaxillary force applied to wired splints. Tantalum implants were placed prior to the experimental period which ranged from 6 to 12 weeks. Serial cephalometric radiographs, *in vivo* bone marking and histology were used in the evaluation of the treatment effect.
Findings: Although there were marked dentofacial changes, particularly at the sutures, the minor nature of the remodelling changes at the temporomandibular joint did not support the concept that skeletal malocclusion can be corrected by transformation of the joint in the adult.

Mills, J.R.E. (1978) The effects of orthodontic treatment on the skeletal pattern. *British Journal of Orthodontics*, **5**, 133–143.

A thorough literature review covering the effects of headgear and functional appliances on the skeletal pattern.
Findings: The author concludes that if changes occur they are small in amount and take considerable time to achieve.

Mills, J.R.E. (1983) Clinical control of craniofacial growth — a skeptics viewpoint. In: McNamara, J.A. Jr, Ribbens, K.A. & Howe, R.P. (eds) *Clinical alteration of the growing face*, Monograph 14. Centre for Human Growth and Development, University of Michigan.

This paper contains a detailed appraisal of the published clinical evidence concerning the effect of functional appliances on facial growth.

Findings:
1 The major changes produced by myofunctional appliances are essentially dental in nature.
2 Skeletal changes can be summarized as follows:
(a) Functional appliances produce a reduction in the angle ANB of approximately 1 degree more than would be expected to occur without treatment, but this may not be maintained in the long term.

(b) The length of the mandible increases by 0.5 mm a year more than in control groups but even this small increase is not maintained for long after treatment is finished.

(c) There is an increase in both posterior and anterior face heights with functional treatment which may be maintained in the long term.

3 The suggestion that functional appliance therapy in the growing child is an alternative to orthognathic surgery is grossly optimistic.

Morndall, O. (1984) The effect on the incisor teeth of activator treatment: a follow-up study. *British Journal of Orthodontics*, **11**, 214−220.

A study of the records of 40 Class II division 1 cases treated by the Andresen method. Despite its title the paper is concerned with changes during treatment. Mean age at the start was 11 years and at the end of treatment 12.5 years. In some cases, to avoid labial tipping, acrylic was extended over the lower incisal edges.

Findings: Lower incisors developed more crowding in 12% of cases. In 18% crowding reduced. 25% of all patients showed retroclination of lower incisors during treatment and there was significant negative correlation between pre-treatment and post-treatment angulations.

The author concludes that proclination of the lower incisors is not a contra-indication of treatment with the activator.

Nielsen, I.L. (1984) Facial growth during treatment with the function regulator appliance. *American Journal of Orthodontics*, **85**, 125−134.

This is a report of 10 out of 12 consecutive cases (six girls, four boys, two cases discontinued) treated by the author using the FR2. Superimposition of headfilms was made using stable structures in the anterior cranial base.

Findings:
1 Facial growth changes were mainly in the vertical plane.
2 The maxilla generally became more retrognathic during treatment.
3 In the mandible there was great individual variation but no indication was found that the FR2 promoted forward growth of the mandible.
4 The sagittal improvement seen in occlusion was due more to changes in the vertical plane than to sagittal growth.

Owen, A.H. (1983) Morphologic changes in the transverse dimension using Frankel appliances. *American Journal of Orthodontics*, **83**, 200−217.

An examination of 50 Class I and Class II patients treated with Frankel appliances (mean age of 9.6 years) who gave clinical evidence of good co-operation, of wearing a Frankel appliance 20 hours per day. The Rocky Mountain Data Services growth predictions were used as controls. Evaluation was made from frontal cephalometric radiographs.

Findings: There was a limited but significant increase in nasal cavity width and maxillary and mandibular arch width during treatment compared with RMDS predictions (P < 0.05). No long-term follow-up was made. See also McDougal *et al.* (1982).

Owen, A.H. (1986) Maxillary incisolabial responses in Class II Division 1 treatment with Frankel and Edgewise. *Angle Orthodontist*, **56**, 67−87.

Fifty patients (26 female, 24 male) treated with the Frankel appliance were compared with 50 (25 male, 25 female) treated with the Edgewise appliance. In the later group 33 wore headgear, 16 had four first premolars extracted and six upper first premolars only.

From his cephalometric study this author concludes that:
1 Frankel treatment tends to retract the maxillary incisors less than the Edgewise appliance.
2 Frankel treatment tends to retract the A-point less than multibanded therapy.
3 The upper lip tends to move forward with Frankel treatment, but backwards with fixed appliance therapy during overjet correction.
4 The naso-labial angle tends to become more obtuse during Edgewise treatment, but remain at near the pre-treatment value with Frankel treatment.

Owen, A.H. (1988) Frontal facial changes with the Frankel appliance. *Angle Orthodontist*, **58**, 257−287.

Fifty patients treated with the Frankel appliance (26 girls, 24 boys, mean age 9.6 years, range 5.9−13.8 years) were compared with 50 patients treated successfully with Edgewise mechanics. Both Class I and Class II molar cases were included. Using pre and post treatment cephalometric PA skull radiographs, the author found that there was a significantly greater increase in the bigonial dimension in the Frankel group when compared with the controls drawn from the Foundation for Orthodontic Research and Bolton Studies.

Pancherz, H. (1976) Long term effects of activator (Andresen appliance) treatment. *Odontologisk Revy*, **27** (Suppl. 35), 11−42.

From a total of 142 patients treated with activators constructed according to Andresen, 112 were followed up for between 10 and 20 years. Only 58 had pre-treatment, post-treatment and follow-up radiographs. Of these 34 had also received extractions of premolars or molars. Electromyographic records were obtained for 19 patients.

Findings:
1 Lower incisors continued to procline throughout the treatment and follow-up period but when lower incisor angulation was measured with respect to the sella-nasion line no significant changes were found.
2 There was a continuous reduction in arch length during and after treatment. At follow-up 93% of maxillary extraction spaces and 85% of mandibular extraction spaces had closed. During the follow-up period 26% of extraction cases and 23% of non-extraction cases showed an increase in crowding.
3 EMG results demonstrated that activator treatment does not result in the formation of a 'dual bite' and there was no greater incidence in symptoms of mandibular dysfunction than in untreated subjects.
4 The angulation of teeth adjacent to the extraction sites showed continued improvement during the follow-up period.

Pancherz, H. (1977) Relapse after activator treatment: a biometric, cephalometric and electromyographic study of subjects with and without relapse of overjet. *American Journal of Orthodontics*, **72**, 499−512.

A report of 19 patients 10–20 years after treatment. Cephalograms, EMG studies and models were used in the evaluation. EMGs were only recorded following treatment.

Findings:
1 An openbite following treatment was associated with relapse.
2 There was a greater increase in the intercanine width in the stable group.
3 ANB was greater before and after treatment in the relapsed group.
4 There was an increase in the MM angle in the relapsed group.
5 Mentalis activity was greater in the relapsed group.
  Conclusion: relapse is associated with adverse growth and adverse tongue activity.

Pancherz, H. (1981) The effect of continuous bite jumping on the dento-facial complex: a follow-up study after Herbst appliance treatment of Class II malocclusion. *European Journal of Orthodontics*, **3**, 49–60.

The effects of the Herbst appliance were investigated in ten consecutively treated boys with Class II division 1 malocclusions examined one year after treatment. These were compared with changes seen in ten untreated controls of the same age and sex.

Findings:
1 The influence of the appliance on maxillary growth appeared to be reversible.
2 Sagittal mandibular growth was accelerated during treatment. No adverse changes were seen during the 12-month follow-up.

Pancherz, H. (1984) A cephalometric analysis of skeletal changes contributing to Class II correction in activator treatment. *American Journal of Orthodontics*, **85**, 125–134.

Cephalometric changes of 30 successfully treated Class II division 1 cases were analysed using a superimposition on anterior cranial base structures. Treatment changes were compared with Bolton standards for persons exhibiting excellent occlusion.

Findings:
1 Improvement in incisor and molar occlusion was about equally attributable to dental and skeletal changes.
2 The average overjet reduction of 5.0 mm was produced by 2.4 mm of relative mandibular growth and 2.5 mm distal movement of the maxillary incisors but only 0.1 mm of mesial movement of the lower incisors.
3 When the findings were compared to the Bolton standards the treatment appeared to have:
  (a) inhibited maxillary growth;
  (b) moved the maxillary incisors and molars distally;
  (c) moved the mandibular incisors and molars mesially.
There was no apparent affect on mandibular growth.

Pancherz, H., Hansen K. (1988) Mandibular anchorage in Herbst treatment. *European Journal of Orthodontics*, **10**, 149–164.

This investigation was undertaken to determine the efficiency of five mandibular anchorage systems in Herbst treatment of 65 Class II division 1 cases by measuring the extent to which lower incisors proclined. Treatment on average lasted 7 months and follow-up was undertaken at 6 and 12 months post treatment.

It was found that none of the systems could eliminate anterior movement of incisors and molars but that 80% of the incisor movement and 20% of the molar movement recovered after treatment. Although the authors conclude that post treatment changes in tooth position did not contribute to lower incisor crowding, there was pretreatment spacing of 0.6 mm (SD 1.1 mm) in the mandibular incisor segment and illustrations suggest that some cases also had spacing in the buccal segments.

Pancherz, H. & Harsen, K. (1986) Occlusal changes during and after Herbst treatment: a cephalometric investigation. *European Journal of Orthodontics* **8**, 215–228.

Changes during and after Herbst treatment were investigated in 40 subjects who had Class II division 1 malocclusions. During an average of 7 months treatment all cases achieved Class I or Class III arch relationships. In the 12-month period following treatment the occlusion settled into Class I in all cases. About 90% of the occlusal relapse occurred in the first 6 months. In 58% of cases this was exclusively the result of tooth movement but unfavourable maxillary–mandibular growth contributed to the occlusal relapse in 17 cases.

Post-treatment retention and occlusal adjustment are recommended with this type of treatment.

Pancherz, H. & Pancherz-Anehus, M. (1982) The effect of continuous bite jumping with the Herbst appliance on the masticatory system: a functional analysis. *European Journal of Orthodontics*, **4**, 37–44.

The functional effects of the Herbst appliance were investigated electromyographically and by means of clinical tests in 20 boys with Class II division 1 malocclusions.

Findings: Treatment with the Herbst appliance resulted in minor functional disturbances which appeared mainly at the beginning of treatment and were of a temporary nature.

Parkhouse, R.C. (1968) Cephalometric appraisal of cases of Angles Class II division 1 malocclusion treated by the Andresen appliance. *Transactions of the British Society for the Study of Orthodontics*, **55**, 61–70.

Forty-six Class II division 1 cases in which Andresen appliances had been used were compared to 30 control cases in which similar malocclusions had received various treatments, some including upper arch extractions. In the experimental group both successful and unsuccessful cases were included.

Findings: Over a period of 3 years 2 months the Andresen treated patients showed a favourable change of 1.5 mm in forward movement of the B-point but this is derived from an SNB angular change of less than 1 degree. Good co-operation achieved a greater mean SNB change than bad, although differences were small and treatment times not comparable.

Petrovic, A., Stutzman, B., Ozerovic, B. & Vidovic, Z. (1982) Does the Frankel appliance produce forward movement of mandibular premolars? *European Journal of Orthodontics*, **4**, 173–183.

Tissue culture techniques were used to detect the site and rate of formation of bone in the mandibular premolar region following 3 weeks treatment with the Frankel appliance. The sample consisted of 45 11–13 year-old boys with Class II division 1 malocclusions. Nineteen showed forward growth rotation of the mandible and 26 backward rotation.

Findings: The functional regulator does not promote mesially directed movement of the mandibular premolars but instead tends to encourage increased premolar eruption. The authors note that the clinical effectiveness of the appliance was greater in patients who had anterior patterns of mandibular growth rotation.

Pfeiffer, J.P. & Grobety, D. (1982) A philosophy of combined orthopaedic orthodontic treatment. *American Journal of Orthodontics*, **81**, 185–201.

Essentially this is a descriptive paper on the uses of the activator of the Harvold type with headgear to the upper and reverse headgear to the lower arch where appropriate. Treatment is started early, before the growth spurt.

Reey, R.W. & Eastwood, A. (1978) The passive activator: case selection, treatment response and corrective mechanisms. *American Journal of Orthodontics*, **73**, 378–409.

An interesting description of the authors' design of activator which has features common to both the Harvold and Andresen/Haupl patterns.

A study of 31 Class II division 1 cases is included in which cephalometric changes are compared with the growth changes predicted by Rocky Mountain Data Systems.

Robertson, N.R.E. (1983) An examination of treatment changes in children treated with the function regulator of Frankel. *American Journal of Orthodontics*, **83**, 299–310.

The cephalometric changes seen in two groups of 12 subjects whose uncrowded Class II and Class III malocclusions treated by means of the function regulator were examined using the Ricketts 10-factor analysis. The results were compared to values obtained from Michigan growth study data.

Findings:
1 In the Class II group the incisor correction was achieved by a combination of palatal tipping of the upper incisors together with some proclination of the lower incisors. In the Class III group correction was primarily the result of lower incisor retroclination.
2 Skeletal as distinct from dento-alveolar changes were minimal.

Schmuth, G.P.F. (1983) Milestones in the development and practical application of functional appliances. *American Journal of Orthodontics*, **84**, 48–53.

This is a brief but interesting account of the development and use of functional appliances.

Stockli, P.W. & Deitrich, U.C. (1973) Experimental and clinical findings following functional forward displacement of the mandible. *Transactions of the European Orthodontic Society and Third International Orthodontic Congress*, 435–442.

The paper has two parts. In the first histological evaluation of the condylar and glenoid fossa structures of six macaque monkeys supports the view that the condyle and glenoid fossa show compensatory tissue reactions when the mandible is held 5 mm in front of centric jaw relationship. The second is an examination of the cephalometric records of 25 patients with Class II division 1 malocclusions treated by use of the activator. This failed to demonstrate any treatment-induced anterior development of the mandible.

Teuscher, U. (1978) A growth related concept for skeletal Class II treatment. *American Journal of Orthodontics*, **74**, 258–275.

A case is put forward for the use of an activator with minimal bite opening with high pull headgear applied through tubes attached to the activator.

Tomer, B.S. & Harvold, E.P. (1982) Primate experiments on mandibular growth direction. *American Journal of Orthodontics*, **82**, 114–119.

Sixteen Rhesus monkeys implanted with stainless steel markers were used to investigate the effect of nasal obstruction on mandibular growth. Cephalometric radiographs and models were taken at 3-month intervals throughout the 3-year experiment.

Findings: The authors found that animals in the experimental group developed increased facial height, steeper mandibular planes and increased gonial angles. Since the ramus of the mandible retained its shape in the experimental animals the authors concluded that the muscles of mastication were not significantly affected and that the ramus/masticatory muscles and chin/suprahyoid, orofacial muscle are two relatively independent systems.

Trayfoot, J. & Richardson, A. (1968) Angle Class II division 1 malocclusion treated by the Andresen method: An analysis of 17 cases. *British Dental Journal*, **124**, 516–519.

Eight male and nine female patients with Class II division 1 malocclusions treated with an Andresen appliance were matched with 17 similar controls.

Findings:
1 That SNA and SNB changed significantly due to the reduction of SNA and an increase in SNB.
2 The correction was due more to maxillary restriction than 'mandibular growth'.
3 Forward movement of B-point, although twice that observed in the controls, was small (0.97 degree).

Valant, R.J. & Sinclair, P.M. (1989) Treatment effects of the Herbst appliance. *American Journal of Orthodontics*, **95**, 138–147.

Thirty-two consecutively treated Herbst appliance patients with Class II division 1 malocclusions (14 male, 18 female, mean age 10 years 2 months) were compared with a control group drawn from the Michigan Growth Study. (Unfortunately this was signficantly less Class II in terms of angle ANB than the experimental group.)

The authors conclude that, in comparison with the controls, Class II correction had been achieved by:
1 An average of 1.5 mm greater forward mandibular growth with a minimum of inhibition of maxillary forward growth.
2 A slight bodily forward movement of the lower incisors but no significant change in the position of the upper incisors.

Vargervik, K. & Harvold, E.P. (1985) Response to activator treatment in Class II malocclusion. *American Journal of Orthodontics*, **88**, 242–251.

Activators of the Harvold pattern were used in the treatment of 85 subjects with Class II malocclusion in the mixed dentition stage. Cephalometric comparisons were made between the changes which were observed in each 6-month increment of the treatment period (mean 35 months). In half the subjects comparison was made between treatment changes and those in the pre-treatment period. In 18 subjects post-treatment comparisons were also possible.

Findings:
1 There was significant reduction in forward growth of the maxilla and the usual dental changes (reduction of the overjet, levelling of the occlusal planes, improved molar relationship).
2 There was no conclusive evidence that the mandibular length was increased by treatment but some suggestion that the glenoid fossa became more inferiorly and anteriorly located.
3 Because the slight inhibition of the maxilla and relocation of the glenoid fossa seen in the longitudinal study could not account for the correction of the Class II relationship the authors conclude that smaller changes occurred at other sites which were insufficiently marked to reach statistical significance.

Note: As the authors point out, the 'controls' were the same subjects in the pre- and post-treatment period. Differences between growth rates in the treatment and control periods could therefore be due to the effects of growth spurts.

Watson, W.G. (1982) Editorial: functional appliances questioned. *American Journal of Orthodontics*, **82**, 519–521.

This is a good conservative view of the state of clinical practice and clinical research in relation to functional appliance therapy.

Wieslander, L. & Lagerstrom, L (1979) The effect of activator treatment in Class II malocclusions. *American Journal of Orthodontics*, **75**, 20–26.

Thirty patients who had responded well to activator treatment carried out during the mixed dentition were compared with a matched group of Class II controls.

All activators were constructed according to the principles of Andresen.

Findings:
1 The effect of treatment was usually of dento-alveolar origin.
2 Although the lower incisors were intruded they were not significantly protruded.
3 Despite excellent individual responses the average orthopaedic effect was limited.

4 There was a significant increase in the lower face height in the activator group compared with the controls after treatment but no difference 4 years later.
5 There was no significant difference in the amount of mandibular growth seen in the two groups.

Williams, S. & Melsen, B. (1982) Condylar development and mandibular rotation and displacement during activator treatment—an implant study. *American Journal of Orthodontics*, **81**, 322–326.
and
Williams, S. & Melsen, B. (1982) The interplay between sagittal and vertical growth factors—an implant study of activator treatment. *American Journal of Orthodontics*, **81**, 327–332.

This most interesting implant study reported here in two papers examines the interplay of condylar growth, and vertical and horizontal sutural and alveolar growth, during the correction of Class II jaw relationship ($n=19$). Sagittal correction was measured both in terms of the change in the angle ANB and by means of a modified Witts analysis.

Findings:
1 Despite attempts to reduce upper molar eruption by use of lateral bite planes, vertical dento-alveolar growth was pronounced in the maxillary molar region (only a low construction bite was used).
2 The most important determinants of changes in the sagittal jaw relationship were posterior maxillary vertical development, vertical condylar growth, sagittal condylar growth and vertical development of the maxillary alveolar process.

The authors conclude that control of the vertical dimension is imperative for optimum forward displacement of the mandible in the correction of Class II skeletal malocclusion.

Woodside, D.G., Metaxis, A. & Altuna, G. (1989) The influence of functional appliance therapy on glenoid fossa remodelling. *American Journal of Orthodontics*, **92**, 181–198.

This is a report of a radiographic implant study of the effect of a 'progressively advanced' Herbst appliance on seven Macaca fascicularis monkeys (7 female, 1 male).

The authors conclude that the mandibular advancement produced extensive remodelling and anterior relocation of the glenoid fossa which contributed to the altered jaw relationship.

Woodside, D.G., Reed, R.T., Doucet, J.D. & Thompson, G.W. (1973) Some effects of activator treatment in the growth rate on the mandible and position of the midface. *Transactions of the European Orthodontic Society and Third International Orthodontic Congress*, 443–447.

A condensed report of four studies into the effect of the activator on the mandibular growth rate, mandibular length and position of the structures of the midface.

There were two experimental groups, one where conventional construction bites had been used ($n=9$) and the other where the opening was 10–15 mm beyond the rest position ($n=10$). These were compared to a control group selected from cases in the Burlington Growth Study using serial 45 degree cephalometric radiographs.

Findings:

1 The activator had no effect on the growth velocity of the mandible or its ultimate length in males. In females there was significantly more growth in the female controls.

2 There was little difference in the two types of activator in restricting forward growth of the midface, but widely opened activators caused a downward displacement of the midface and subspinale.

Woodside, D.G., Altuna, G., Harvold, E., Herbert, M. & Metaxas, A. (1983) Primate experiments in malocclusion and bone induction. *American Journal of Orthodontics*, **83**, 460−468.

This is a review of the authors' continuing primate work on the induction of condylar growth through altered muscle function. From the experiments reported in this paper they conclude:

1 That chronic alteration of mandibular position induces extensive condylar remodelling.

2 Downward and backward rotation of the mandible may produce large increases in the mandibular length.

3 Short periods of induced hyperactivity in the muscles of mastication are associated with the production of long-lasting malocclusion.

4 Muscle activity beyond certain limits may interfere with bone remodelling.

Yemm, R. & Nordstrom, S.H. (1974) Forces developed by tissue elasticity as a determinant on mandibular resting position of the rat. *Archives of Oral Biology*, **19**, 347−351.

Whilst aimed at a prosthetic audience this paper is of interest to orthodontists particularly in dealing with the longer term changes in mandibular rest position and its relationship with lower face height.

Appendix 2   Appliance Construction*

A1 Laboratory procedure for the construction of the activator

Upper and lower models poured from well-extended impressions should be supplied, together with a wax working bite. Duplicate the models prior to construction: this will assist the technician in the final trimming of the appliance.

The original models with the wax bite in place are mounted on a plane line articulator. Accurate seating of the bite is crucial at this stage, otherwise the appliance will be constructed to an incorrect bite (Fig. A1.1). If the models are mounted sideways construction of the wire work and fabrication of the acrylic work will be made easier as the vertical arm of the articulator will no longer be an obstruction. The screw setting on the articulator is adjusted and firmly locked after which the wax bite can be discarded.

In order to permit vertical growth of the posterior teeth and prevent forward movement of the anterior sections, certain areas of the dentition must be relieved. The areas are (Fig. A1.2): (a) upper posteriors; (b) lingual to the upper incisors; (Fig. A1.3) (a) lower posteriors, (b) lingual to the lower incisors.

The amount of relief is also important, and it can be seen from the illustrations that the lower posterior sections are relieved considerably (Fig. A1.4), whereas only a thin relief is required in the upper, so that the interocclusal shelf of the finished appliance is in contact with the cusps of the upper posterior teeth (Fig. A1.5). Blocking out of the lower incisors is confined to the lingual of $\overline{21/12}$, it is 1 mm thick and extends down on to the soft tissue for approximately 5 mm (Fig. A1.3).

Construction of the labial bow can now proceed, using 0.9-mm stainless steel wire. The bow should enter the interocclusal acrylic between $\underline{43/34}$. The 'U' loops should be a little larger than those of conventional design on removable appliances, but not so deep as to cause discomfort or ulceration to the patient (Fig. A1.6 a and b). To reduce the risk of wire fractures it is accepted practice to reinforce the bow with tubing where it enters the acrylic.

The acrylic work is applied in heat cured, or self-polymerizing (cold-cure) acrylic according to the preference of the clinician. If the heat-cured method is to be used the appliance has to be waxed. The extent of the wax/acrylic is best described as being like an upper and lower appliance joined at the occlusal surface block. The appliance extends to $\underline{6/6}$, $\overline{6/6}$ distally, up to and over occlusal surfaces of the $\underline{654/456}$, $\overline{654/456}$, up to $\underline{321/123}$, incisal tips, and up to and over the $\overline{321/123}$, terminating one-third of the way down the labial surface to form a capping of acrylic. The space between the upper and lower anterior teeth is left open to form a breathing hole. The lower lingual flange is extended well down into the lower lingual sulcus.

If the cold cure method is to be used, wax buccal shields should be fabricated which will act as a 'dam' thus preventing the cold cure running through the interocclusal area and allowing the material to be built up in layers. A wax ledge constructed below the incisal third of $\overline{321/123}$ will also assist the technician when forming the incisor capping.

After polymerization of the acrylic, the appliance should be removed from the models (Fig. A1.7) and finished. Constant reference to the duplicate set of models is necessary to ensure that the appliance is not being overtrimmed.

When satisfied that the appliance has been trimmed correctly it can be polished in all areas except the fitting surfaces. The blocked out acrylic can be polished on the tooth side but only very slightly in the upper posterior regions, as over-enthusiastic polishing in this area will lead to loss of contact with the upper posterior teeth. This completed, the finished appliance is ready for insertion by the orthodontist (Figs A1.8 and A1.9).

To reduce the bulk of the appliance the palatal acrylic can be replaced by an anterior palatal arch.

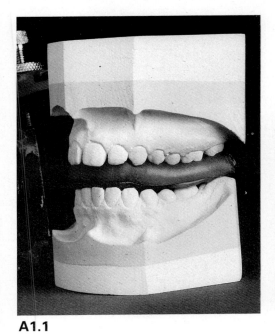

A1.1

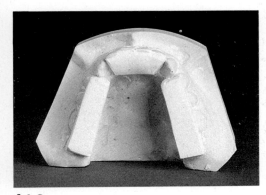

A1.2

A1.3

*The appliances in this section were contructed by J. J. Thompson Ltd, Orthodontic Appliances, 95 Hill Street, Sheffield S2 4SP, Tel: (0742) 759585.

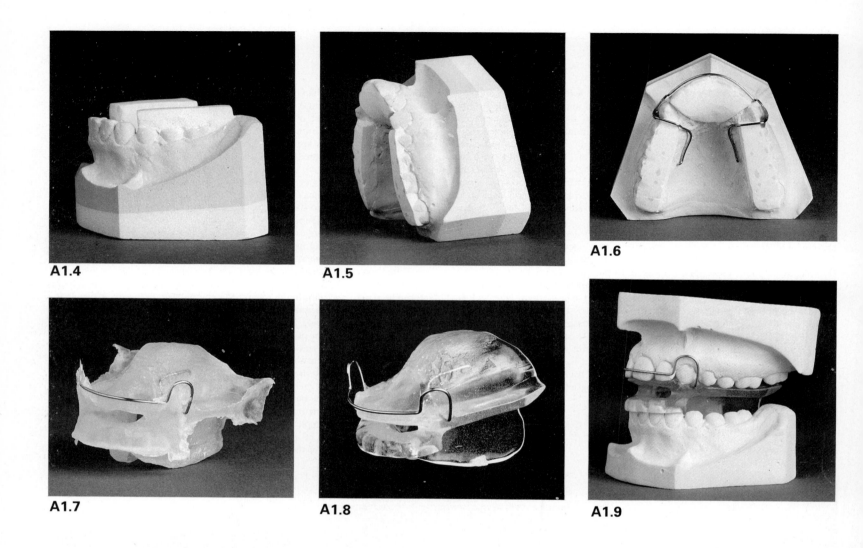

A1.4

A1.5

A1.6

A1.7

A1.8

A1.9

A2 Laboratory procedure for the construction of the Andresen appliance

The procedure for the construction of the Andresen appliance is similar to that of the activator previously described, and the latter can be followed with a few exceptions.

The first point to note is that the dentition is not blocked out. Instead channels (facets) are ground out of the inter-occlusal acrylic to promote downwards and distal movement of the upper posteriors, and upwards and mesial movement of the lower posterior teeth.

The accuracy of the trimming is critical and must be carried out with care. It is important to trim away enough material to allow the vertical movements to take place, but positive contact on the mesio-lingual cusps of 654/456 and disto-lingual

cusps of 654/456 must be maintained to initiate distal (upper) and mesial (lower) movement.

Secondly, although the Andresen is capped in $\overline{321/123}$ area, the acrylic is cut away from 321/123. The labial bow is made from 0.9 mm wire (Figs A2.1 and A2.2) and can be reinforced with tube if required. As the working bites are closer than those of the activator, care should be taken when positioning the labial bow.

Processing is carried out in the usual manner using either heat or self-curing acrylic resin. It is important at the finishing stage not to polish the facets as this will result in loss of tooth contact (Fig. A2.3).

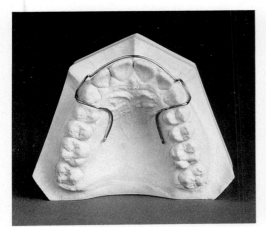

A2.1

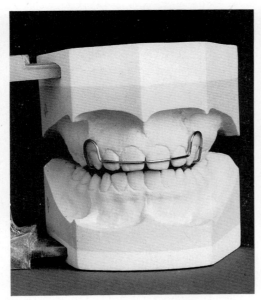

A2.2

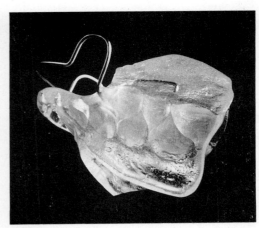

A2.3

A3 Laboratory procedure for the construction of the twin block appliance

Upper and lower models with the working wax bite in place are mounted on a plane line articulator. To facilitate ease of construction the articulator arms are oiled slightly, allowing the models to slide off (Fig. A3.1).

The twin block consists of upper and lower removable appliances. The wire components consist of Adams clasps in 0.7 mm stainless steel wire on 65/56 or 6/6 if the second premolars are not present; a labial bow (0.7 mm) embraces 3/3 (Fig. A3.2); in the lower, Adams clasps 6/6 and a Southend clasp 1/1, all in 0.7-mm wire (Fig. A3.3).

The bridges of the Adams clasps in the upper have a series of coils built into their construction which receive the extra-oral bow. The tubes are made by coiling the 0.7-mm wire around a length of 1.25-mm wire. Six or eight coils will give adequate tube length with a large enough internal diameter to house the EOT bow.

In our experience it is better to heat cure the appliance as it is easier and more accurate to construct the inclined planes. Having completed the wire work, the models are returned to the articulator before being waxed up. The lower blocks are made to cover the occlusal surfaces of 54/45 with the distal edge angled at 45 degrees and terminating distal to 5/5. Extend the wax work up to the lower incisors to form capping over 321/123.

The upper molar blocks cover the occlusal surfaces of 65/56, the mesial edge angled to conform exactly with the lower block. Exact contact is best achieved by occluding the upper and lower models when the upper molar block wax is still soft. The angle of the lower will be reproduced in the soft wax ensuring smooth contact.

The appliances are flasked, packed and finished using conventional methods. When finishing the appliances be very careful not to erode the angles in the molar blocks (Fig. A3.7).

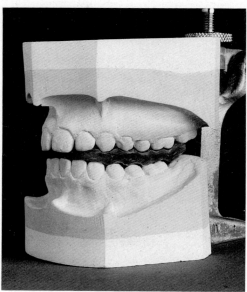

A3.1

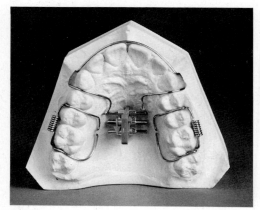

A3.2

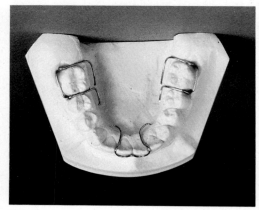

A3.3

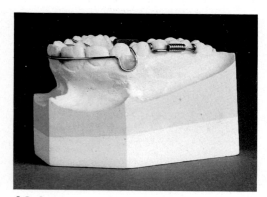

A3.4

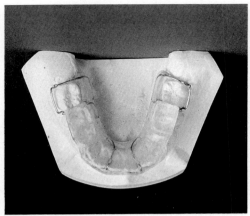

A3.5

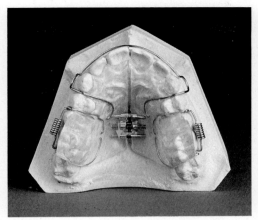

A3.6

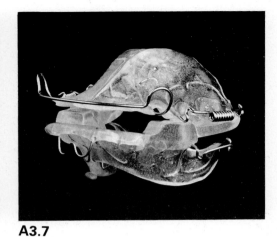

A3.7

A4 Laboratory procedure for the construction of the function regulator

Upper and lower models, cast from well-extended impressions, are mounted with the wax working bite in place, on a plane line articulator. The articulator screw is firmly set after which the wax bite may be discarded.

Construction begins with the fabrication of wax spacers for the buccal regions of the upper and lower models. The purpose of the spacers is to create space between the acrylic buccal shields of the Frankel and the dentition. The technician will find it helpful if the models are removed from the articulator at this stage. To this end it is advisable when mounting the models to oil lightly the arms of the articulator.

Wax is built up in layers starting in the area of the 3/3, $\overline{3/3}$ and extending posteriorly to the posterior border. It is extended occlusally beyond the surfaces of the posteriors, so the upper spacers meet with their lower counterparts inter-occlusally, and in the other direction vertically, terminating at the sulcus. The thickness of the wax spacers is usually about 3 mm (Figs A4.1 and A4.2). Another spacer (thinner than the buccal ones) is constructed in the lower labial area below the gingival margin of the lower anteriors and extending to the sulcus. This is to create space between the lip pad and the gum work, and should be about 1 mm thick (Fig. A4.3).

Having completed the spacers, reassemble the models on to the articulator and check that the bite has not been inadvertently opened by the spacers. If it has, some trimming of the wax will be necessary.

The wire components are constructed from 0.9-mm-diameter stainless steel wire. The models may once again be removed to allow the wire work to proceed unhindered. The lower hangers are the first components to be made. These pass occlusally between $\overline{65/56}$, extend two-thirds into the lingual sulcus area, and on the buccal side down one-third into the sulcus, turning distally and terminating on the posterior border of the model (Figs A4.4 and A4.5).

Next, the lower lingual flange is poured using self-curing acrylic. This is trimmed, polished, refitted to the model and held in position with wax. The lip pads supporting wires are now made and held in position in the fraenum and $\overline{3/3}$ areas with wax (Figs A4.6 and A4.7).

The palatal bow is now constructed. This passes occlusally mesial to 6/6 and then runs two-thirds of the way into the sulcus, returning to form occlusal rests on 6/6 (Fig. A4.8). The canine loops extend two-thirds around the labial surface of 3/3, form a palatal loop and then pass bucally distal to the canines, to terminate on the surface of the wax spacers (Fig. A4.9).

The labial bow touches 21/12, extends downwards and posteriorly into the sulcus, terminating on the outer surface of the spacers (Fig. A4.10). All the wire should have a slight clearance under which the acrylic can flow.

The models are now returned to the articulator and the wax spacers sealed together with a hot knife. Isolating wax is used to outline the shape of the buccal shields and lip pads (Figs A4.11 and A4.12). Self-curing acrylic is applied in layers to form buccal shields and lip pads. It must cover the full extent of the spacers and extend up to the sulci and isolating wax. After sufficient acrylic has been added to cover the wire components, polymerization should be undertaken using a pressure vessel.

The polymerized appliance is then removed from its models and all wax removed. It is trimmed to the required shape, outlined by the isolating wax and the shape of the sulcus. Sufficient clearance should be given to all muscle attachments. The outer surfaces of the acrylic are polished and particular attention should be given to the edges of the buccal shields and lip pads as they should be well rounded for the patient's comfort.

This appliance is fragile and easily distorted, therefore great care should be exercised when polishing.

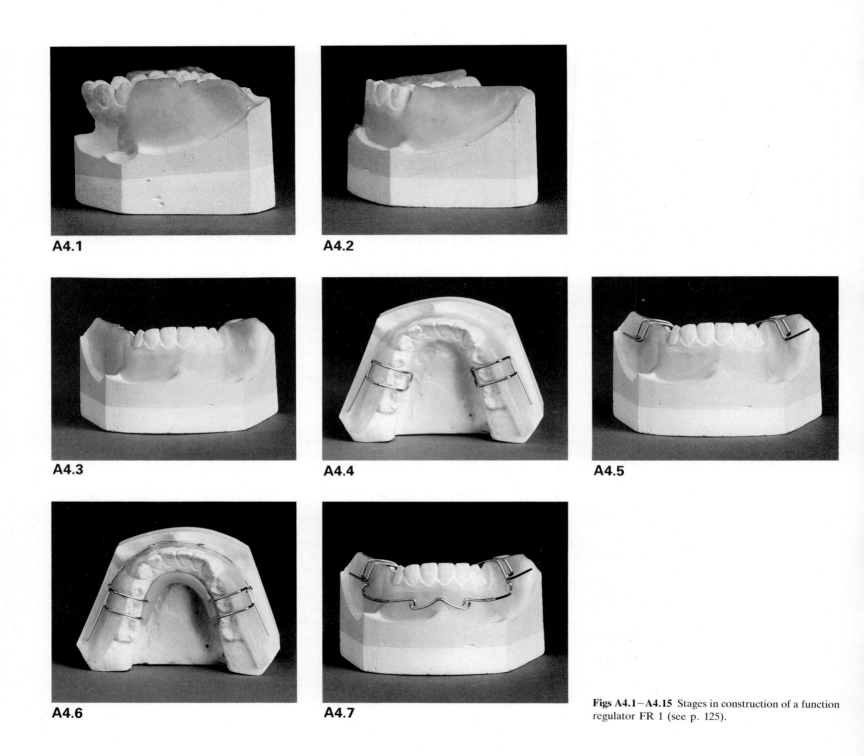

A4.1

A4.2

A4.3

A4.4

A4.5

A4.6

A4.7

Figs A4.1−A4.15 Stages in construction of a function regulator FR 1 (see p. 125).

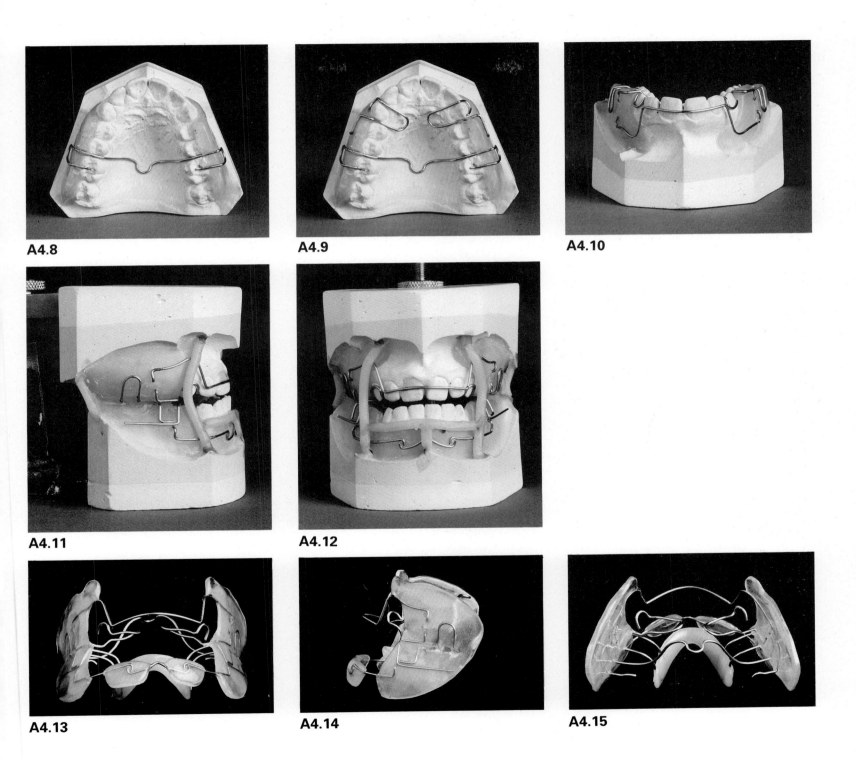

A4.8

A4.9

A4.10

A4.11

A4.12

A4.13

A4.14

A4.15

Index